Praise for *Help Heal Yourself from Cancer*

"This new book by Dr. Bill and Martha Sears provides practical advice and guidance for patients with cancer and their families on how to embark on the journey to heal from cancer. The book is a riveting read that empowers patients and their families with self-help tools to become wiser partners in their cancer care."

—Mahtab Jafari, PharmD, author of *The Truth About Dietary Supplements*, and professor of pharmaceutical sciences at the University of California, Irvine

"We are all blessed with a powerful God-given immune system, but most don't give it that much thought or attention. Using Lifestyle, Exercise, Attitude, and Nutrition—something Dr. Bill and Martha Sears refer to as 'L.E.A.N.'—you can empower your immune army to stay on alert and prevent good cells from turning bad. This book will teach you how to work smarter with your doctor, customize an action plan, and take charge of your recovery by using invaluable, empowering, enlightening concepts such as 'your genes are not your destiny,' 'your soil is more important than your seeds,' and 'you're not a statistic or a percentage.' Healing takes courage, and we all have courage, even if we have to dig deep to find it. To find the courage you need to heal from cancer, just turn the page!"

—Bryce Wylde, DHMHS, functional medicine clinician, founder of Mymmunity, cofounder of The DNA Company

"*Help Heal Yourself from Cancer* empowers each of us to take control of our health and healthcare, with practical insight to help patients through their cancer healing journey. In an easy-to-read-and-understand format, important features of the book include practical science-based tips and guidance for building a conquer-cancer diet, building and partnering with your conquer-cancer team, and living 'L.E.A.N.' This is a must-read, serving as a guide for both patients and their health care team."

—Marla Anderson, MD, FACS, medical director of surgical breast oncology for Mission Hospital

Help Heal Yourself from Cancer

Also by William Sears, MD

The Dr. Sears T5 Wellness Plan
The Healthy Brain Book

Help Heal Yourself from Cancer

Partner Smarter with Your Doctor,
Personalize Your Treatment Plan,
and Take Charge of Your Recovery

WILLIAM SEARS, MD, and MARTHA SEARS, RN

BenBella Books, Inc.
Dallas, TX

Help Heal Yourself from Cancer copyright © 2022 by William Sears and Martha Sears

BenBella Books, Inc.
10440 N. Central Expressway
Suite 800
Dallas, TX 75231
benbellabooks.com
Send feedback to feedback@benbellabooks.com

BenBella is a federally registered trademark.

Printed in the United States of America
10 9 8 7 6 5 4 3 2 1

Library of Congress Control Number: 2022013293
ISBN 9781637741443 (hardcover)
ISBN 9781637741450 (electronic)

Editing by Leah Wilson
Copyediting by Elizabeth Degenhard
Proofreading by Karen Wise and Cape Cod Compositors, Inc.
Indexing by WordCo
Text design and composition by Aaron Edmiston
Cover design by Ty Nowicki
Printed by Lake Book Manufacturing

To our eight children, eleven grandchildren, and two great-grandchildren:
You all are the precious gifts we have to live for.

Contents

Part II: How to Wisely Partner with Your Cancer-Care Providers

Part III: How to L.E.A.N. into Cancer Healing

Part IV: Top Tips to Conquer Colon, Breast, Brain, and Lung Cancers

Consult Your Doctor First

While the tools in this book help prevent *all* cancers and help *most* cancers heal, you may have special medical circumstances that require you to personalize the self-help portion of our cancer-healing plan. For this reason, *always check with your cancer specialist* before using any of the tools in this book. Remember our mission: to help you wisely partner with your doctor's prescribed treatment.

A Note to Cancer-Care Providers on How to Best Use This Book

Most of today's cancer patients want to be better informed and are motivated to empower themselves with self-help tools. Yet many are also overloaded with internet misinformation and unscientific advice, and vulnerable to trying unproven "alternatives." This book is meant to partner with you in helping your patients with cancer. Our wish is that as you announce your cancer-treatment plan, you will also prescribe to your patients: "Here's your guide-book for conquering cancer and helping yourself heal."

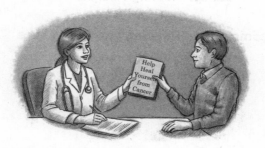

Foreword

As a cancer physician and director of a National Cancer Institute–designated comprehensive cancer center, I have seen firsthand how devastating it is for a patient to be told that they have cancer. Foremost among the emotions that a cancer patient experiences is a feeling of hopelessness, the perception that they have lost control of their health and their lives, which are now in the hands of the medical establishment. Nothing could be further from the truth.

In this excellent guide, Dr. William Sears and his wife Martha Sears, RN, provide an evidence-based roadmap to help patients with cancer, and anyone who wants to avoid getting cancer, take back the reins and become an active participant, together with their health professionals, in the quest to restore and maintain their health. They explore the impact of lifestyle, diet, exercise, and sleep on the body's intrinsic and powerful ability to fight cancer, highlighting the important role of natural killer cells (your "immune system army"). Just as important, they emphasize a positive mindset, spirituality, and managing stress, which we know have major impacts on an individual's response to cancer treatment. Finally, they provide excellent recommendations for how to partner with your oncologist and other cancer care providers. (One of the most important enabling decisions a cancer patient can make is to participate in a clinical trial, where they can help move cancer treatment forward and become a cancer researcher themselves by reporting their personal experiences and outcomes.)

I hope that both lay people and health professionals find this book helpful in maintaining health and navigating the complicated journey that cancer patients find themselves on today. There are many ways to "conquer" cancer, only one of which is to be cured of the disease. The information and suggestions herein can help make that voyage more enlightening, empowering, and emotionally positive.

Richard Van Etten, MD, PhD
Director, UCI Chao Family Comprehensive Cancer Center

Healing Words from Dr. Bill and Nurse Martha

Do you have cancer? Do you want to help someone you love heal from cancer? Do you want to prevent yourself and your loved ones from getting cancer? This book is for you!

We wrote this empowering, cancer-conquering book while we both were healing from cancer—Bill from leukemia, Martha from breast cancer. During Dr. Bill's healing from two cancers (chronic myelogenous leukemia in 2020 and colorectal cancer in 1997), and as other members of the Sears family were healing from breast cancer, bone cancer, and brain cancer, he consulted top cancer specialists in top university cancer centers. He studied science-based medical research and listened to—and learned—the secrets of cancer survivors and purpose-driven thrivers. People become passionate about a project when they are experiencing it.

But on this cancer-healing and cancer-learning journey, he realized there was a missing ingredient in the otherwise rapidly advancing science of cancer treatment: how the patient can support their oncologists' expert care. Bill needed to know: "What can *I do* to help myself heal?"

In this book we share what we learned, and what we did to both partner better with our cancer-care providers and support our natural conquer-cancer armies inside. The changes we made to help heal ourselves are also likely to help us enjoy living longer and healthier—and prevent future cancer. Survivors and "thrivers" who have used these tools to heal from cancer are also more likely to enjoy better health in every other area of their bodies.

Now, we're both enjoying not only healthy bodies but also peace of mind, knowing that we learned, and did, all we could to help ourselves heal. "Getting cancer" triggered our total transformation to a better mind and body. Cancer made us change. That's the transformation we also wish for you.

A healing note from our daughter:

Twenty-five years ago, when I was in college, I got a call from my mom: "Hayden," she said, "Dad has colon cancer. It's serious, and you need to come home."

Thank the Lord, Dad did well through the surgery. The hardest part was after that: the chemotherapy, the radiation, literally watching the hero of my life become so burdened. But during that very difficult time in my family's life, something very beautiful started to happen deep inside my dad. Cancer became his passion, his fire, his obsession. He had to figure out how he could heal himself. But even more than that, he wanted to learn how to keep his eight children from ever having to experience cancer themselves.

His dad died from colon cancer, and my mom's mom died of colon cancer, so genetically it appeared we Sears children would be doomed. But the Lord gave us a secret weapon: our dad.

He spent the next few years of his recovery just poring over research journals. Luckily, he was in a position of his career that gave him access to top minds in health and nutrition. He was able to glean science-based tips from all of these resources. He had a new mission, a new passion in life, and he has spent the last twenty-five years of his career sharing with others what he learned for himself. What you get to read here is not only from the mind of a brilliant scientist, but also from the heart of a father.

Love you, Daddy.

Hayden Sears

How to Get the Most Healing from This Book

Everyone's cancer is unique. How your body fights and heals from cancer is unique. Ponder the following to get the cancer-healing plan that works best for you.

> **You are a partner, not just a patient.**

1. Personalize your pills-plus-skills plan. While you will read and hear the survival "percentage" for your cancer treatment, also remember: *you are a person, not a percentage.* Modern cancer treatment is the best it's ever been, with exciting new treatments such as targeted chemotherapy. And cancer-care providers know more now than ever about how to personalize cancer treatment to the individual.

The treatment prescribed by your cancer-care providers is the *pills* part of your personal cancer healing plan. But remember: *You are a partner, not just a patient.* The self-help *skills* that you will learn in this book—many of which help your doctor-prescribed pills work better——make you a key participant in your cancer-healing team. Select the cancer-conquering tools we provide that most fit *you*. Modify them to better fit you. Then, in partnership with your cancer-care providers, formulate your personalized cancer-healing toolbox that will become part of "you" for the rest of your life.

> Enjoy a "pills–skills" mindset.

2. Enjoy your carry-over effect. Cancer, like many other illnesses, is an *immune system imbalance*. The self-help tools you will learn in Part III of this book to prevent and heal from cancer also help fight nearly all other ailments.

The same tools you will use to heal from cancer also help prevent most other illnesses, especially cardiovascular disease, autoimmune disorders (all those "-itises"), and neuroinflammation disorders responsible for the epidemic of mental unwellness. For nearly all ailments at all ages, Part III is your personal toolbox for healthy living.

Reading, doing, and feeling our conquer-cancer plan will be your *new normal*, and the healing it brings will carry over into the rest of your life. You will notice that, in this book, we purposely use the deeper word *transformation* more than *change*. Transformation is an *inside job*, as is cancer. You will change your biochemistry at the molecular and cellular level, where true health begins and remains.

3. Be peaceful. Many people with cancer go on to experience "decision regrets" or "treatment anxiety": "Oh, I should have done this, and not done that," and so on. Learning and doing our conquer-cancer self-help tools can give you the peace of mind that you are doing the best you can with the information you have. Therefore, no peace-disturbing!

When someone gets a cancer diagnosis, "I'm afraid of . . ." is a usual feeling. Our top wish for our readers is that they are able to quickly shift from a fearful mindset to a healing one. Fear sabotages wise decision-making, and your healing path will be loaded with decisions. This fear factor is why, in Part I, we show you how to shift to, and stay in, a conquer-cancer mindset.

4. Don't play the blame game. Naturally, you may be wondering: "What *caused* my cancer?" For most of us it's not one simple cause but rather an *accumulation* of carcinogens (cancer seeds) that eventually overwhelm our natural conquer-cancer army, the immune system. That's why we are careful to use the term "contributor" to cancer rather than "cause" of cancer. Years and years of many carcinogens gradually add up, and eventually you "get cancer."

Please don't beat yourself up or falsely believe that you got cancer because you weren't already doing all these cancer-healing tips—or if you aren't healing well despite doing them. Many of the carcinogen studies are statistical. You are an individual. It's unlikely you "caused" your cancer by what you ate, didn't eat, stressed about, and other contributors. Go forward with a positive conquer-cancer mindset and don't waste fruitless energy on "I should have . . ." Don't play the blame game. It is so easy to fall into an "if only" pattern of thinking.

And remember: Just as cancer contributors have a *cumulative effect*, so do cancer-healing tools. Research shows that the *more of our self-help tools you use* and the longer you use them, the greater your chances of healing from (and preventing future) cancer.

5. Read wisely. To get the most healing from our book, learn to read much like you will learn how to eat—small, frequent feedings, and small, frequent readings.

Read in real sunlight. To remember and personalize what you read, instead of reading an electronic version, first read the real pages in real light. Because your eyes are windows to your brain, research shows that most people remember and do more of what they read when they read it on paper, in sunlight, than when they read an electronic version in artificial lighting.

Read and reflect. Just hearing the "C-word" is bound to stress you out. So, we want each page—what you see and read with your eyes and mind—to both relax you and inform you. Read a paragraph, look at the illustration, and then take a few minutes to ponder what you read and saw. In fact, each page is purposely designed to help what you read imprint deep in your mind. Follow our formula: read it, learn it, do it, and feel it. Focus more on *what you can do* than the cancer inside you.

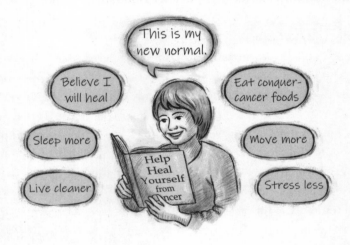

Your cancer can be your great motivator for *change*. You can control it. Or it can control you. Your choice!

Download Your Reminders

You can download many of the tips found throughout this book at AskDrSears.com/cancer-healing. Hang these prompts throughout your home and workplace. Share them with loved ones as constant reminders to keep you on your new path to transformation and healing.

Build Your Cancer-Healing Library

Stay up to date on cancer-healing updates. Since science continues to discover new breakthroughs in prevention and treatment for cancer, see AskDrSears.com/cancer.

Read our cancer-healing partner books.

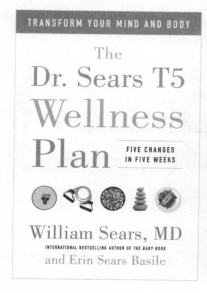
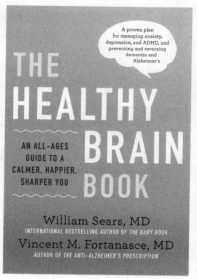

Smartening your conquer-cancer mind begins in your brain. So does building your anti-cancer army: the brain is the commander-in-chief of your immune system. Because the better your brain, the better you heal from cancer, read *The Healthy Brain Book* along with this book to help you go deeper into each cancer-healing tool you will learn to use.

See our suggested cancer-healing library (pages 215–216).

Your conquer-cancer prescription

℞ Sears Family Medicine
7 Cancer Way
Everywhere, USA

- Believe in your body and your immune system army
- Wisely partner with your cancer-care providers
- Eat our conquer-cancer diet
- Move more, sit less, heal better
- Stress less, sick less
- Sleep cancer away

Refills: <u>Forever</u>   <u>William Sears</u> MD

Part I

How to Have a
Conquer-Cancer
Mindset

Cancer healing begins in your brain. As you will now learn, having a conquer-cancer mindset means flooding your brain with those thoughts that prompt your body to heal—thoughts that focus more on the healing tools you have, dwelling more on what *you can do* rather than the disease inside you. We will show you how to master your conquer-cancer mindset by automatically pondering: "Will this food, thought, or action feed or fight my cancer?"

Chapter 1

. . . .

Believe You Will Heal

A top teaching in brain health that sums up our conquer-cancer mindset is:

> **Where attention flows, brain tissue grows.**

Suppose you spend most of your day internally focusing on "I believe I can heal," "My beautiful body can beat this cancer," and other positive prompts. Gradually, you grow more cerebral real estate that reflects on and replays these beliefs. You grow your belief center and shrink your worry center.

The reverse can also happen. Dwelling on fearful thoughts can grow your worry center instead of your belief center.

Which mindset do you want to grow in your brain?

Positivity promotes longevity. A "positive person" is more likely to have planted more positive thoughts into their brain tissue garden. This mindset literally sets you up to make wiser decisions in personalizing your cancer healing journey. We go deeper into this evolving science of *psycho-oncology* (think-changing your brain to make wiser conquer-cancer choices) in Chapter 7.

Cancer healing begins in your mind. Your mindset prompts your brain (the commander of your natural immune system army, or ISA) to fight cancer. The stronger you believe you will heal, the more likely you are to heal. Believers are more likely to become survivors. The more you "put your mind to it" and stay in the "right frame of mind," the better your immune system will work. Your journey to healing from cancer begins with the *belief you will heal* being deeply imprinted into your CCM (conquer-cancer mindset). (In the next chapter you will learn even more about the *belief effect* influencing how smartly your ISA fights your cancer.)

This is why we start this book with how to develop a conquer-cancer mindset. Neuroscientists have long known that optimists, the "don't worry, be happy" crowd, usually get less cancer and heal better than pessimists.

Science supports the conquer-cancer mind. A new specialty in psychiatry, *psycho-oncology*, studies how your mind can affect healing from cancer and other major illnesses. A branch of this field called *psychoneuroimmunology* (PNI) studies how your mind works with your cancer-fighting immune system to fight better for you.

Early on in our healing journeys we studied the secrets of survivors—those who healed from even the most severe illnesses. The top healer that empowered survivors to become thrivers (who not just survived longer but became healthier) was their sincere belief they had what they called a "healer within": a personal conquer-cancer internal medicine pharmacy that was activated by turning their confidence level up a notch.

Fear-Less

Fear fights wise decision-making. A tool for life we teach our kids is: "Don't decide when sad!" In healing from your cancer, you will need clarity of mind to make more wise decisions.

One of the top secrets of survivors is they devote less cerebral real estate to worrying and more to healing. In our healings we upgraded "fear" to F.E.A.R.—*Follow Every Available Resource* that can nourish your healing.

How you open your personal conquer-cancer pharmacy and make it work better for you is still a bit of a medical mystery, yet here's how we think it works. The emerging science of *psychoneuroimmunology* teaches that when your mind believes you will heal, it sends biochemical text messages to your immune system, your natural cancer-fighting army inside, instructing them to fight: "I believe you will heal me. Now go do it!" (See how your immune system fights for you on page 31.)

Another reason believing is healing is that it helps you overcome a cancer-feeding emotion—*loss of control.* Feeling helpless and hopeless depresses your immune system, which in turn impairs its ability to fight.

Believers are more likely to become survivors.

"You've got cancer!" is a mind shock for which you weren't prepared. The more quickly you can shift into a conquer-cancer frame of mind, the more likely you are to heal.

Easier said than done, we know! The cancer-healing mind tools in this chapter will help you quickly upgrade from "Oh no, why me? What should I have done differently?" to "I can beat this!"

Will This Thought, Food, or Action
Feed or *Fight* My Cancer?

Many times a day, before you begin to eat, think, or do something, first ask yourself: Will this food *feed* or *fight* my cancer? (For our conquer-cancer diet, see Chapter 5.) Will this thought *feed* or *fight* my cancer? Will the way I spend my free time *feed* or *fight* my cancer? Imagine your conquer-cancer mind prompting you to "do" or "don't!"

Eventually, you will think-change your mind into *automatically* prompting you on the path to health instead of the path to more cancer. Your "Will this help heal me?" mantra can become your greatest mentor within and carry over to keeping you on your way to a happier and healthier life. Remember a basic fact of brain changing: thoughts change brain structures. Neurologists teach that where thoughts flow, brain tissues grow. Grow your brain's *fight-cancer areas* and shrink your *feed-cancer areas*.

One caveat: The mindset tactic of asking yourself "Will this food, thought, or action feed or fight my *cancer*?" works for some people. Yet, for others, constantly relating everything they think or do to their cancer can become a dysfunctional no-no. It can put them on constant high alert, and make them feel anxious and on edge.

If this is you, instead try focusing your attention on "Will this thought, food, or action feed or fight my *immune system army* (ISA) inside?"

"Dwell" differently. This mindset change, where you dwell more on the powerful ISA inside rather than your cancer, is the new you. When Dr. Bill got the diagnosis "You've got cancer," after a period of dwelling on the cancer inside he realized he was slowly becoming his cancer. He related everything he did to whether it would help or hurt it. After studying and consulting some top neuroscientists, who taught him the principle of "where attention flows, brain tissue grows," he underwent a mindset change. He realized:

Enough! He needed to focus *less on the problem and more on the solution*. Within a few weeks, he was dwelling much more on his healing tools—what he was doing to fight the cancer—and much less on the cancer itself, and he was happier. That's the *transformation* we wish for you.

> Dwell more on what you can do
> than the cancer inside you.

Enjoy More Self-Help Skills to Partner with Your Pills

When your expert cancer doctor prescribes the *pills*—"Here's what you need to *take*" (chemo, radiation, and so on)—naturally, you need to fill in the empowering blank of "Doctor, what can I *do?*"—skills. With most cancers you will need both science-based pills and your own personalized skills. That's our prescription for cancer-healing in a nutshell.

Consider becoming a certified cancer coach. Make learning about cancer-healing your hobby, and get the "helper's high" from sharing what you've learned with others. (See how to become a certified coach, page 46.)

Journal Your Personal Healing Path

Therapeutic writing is a top "medicine" for the Sears family cancer survivors. Cancer specialists have long recognized that people who journal their path heal better. Putting thoughts on paper helps stimulate self-healing thoughts in your mind. It's like sitting down and writing prompts your mind: "Okay, brain, the door is now open to think more clearly. Treasure your thoughts." Write them, read them, practice them, share them!

Writing how you feel and what you did that day to self-heal empowers you to feel more like a partner in your team of healers. In our experience of over fifty years in medical practice, we have noticed—and science confirms—that those who journal their progress feel less helpless and hopeless, and are more likely to stay on their personal path to healing.

> Give your personal cancer-healing journal a fun title, such as *Betty's Beat Breast Cancer Bible.*

Draw your cancer away. Cancer patients who journal their progress and draw their feelings heal better than those who journal alone. It's "art therapy"!

It's also why our cancer-healing book has many times more illustrations than other cancer books. If you see a drawing in this book that rivets your attention, personalize it. Redraw it with your own style and feelings.

Leave a legacy. "Grandpa, what are you writing?" asked our grandchildren.

"How we beat our cancers."

"That's so cool!" they replied.

Fast-forward to your family reading your journal and learning the tools for life you've written for them: make healing your hobby, and take charge of your health.

Listen to the Wisdom of Your Body

At some point in your healing, you will experience a personal dose of the *wisdom of the body*, where your body will let you know what to do to stay on your path to healing.

During his cancer healing, Dr. Bill discovered he had an inner voice that prompted him to eat conquer-cancer foods he'd never thought of eating or didn't previously like, and that waved an internal red flag when he was tempted to eat off the "naughty list." Your body will prompt you—even nag you—on how to heal. You just have to learn to listen to it.

Your "doctors" within. The wisdom of the body is not just about what your body tells you, but about what your body can do. You have four "doctors" within that help you fight cancer:

1. **Your immune system army (ISA).** These are the trillions of pre-trained soldier-cells patrolling your body, ready to kick out those cancer cells. (You will meet your ISA in Chapter 2.)

2. **Your endothelial pharmacy.** The largest "doctor" or healer within your body lies within the lining of your blood vessels, the endothelium, where your body "makes its own medicines" (the trademark teaching of the Dr. Sears Wellness Institute) to help you heal. (You will learn more about this pharmacy, and how to open it, on pages 129–131.)

3. **Your good-gut pharmacy.** Inside the lining of your lower intestines reside trillions more "mini-doctors," called your *microbiome*, the community of bacteria and other organisms that live in the lining of your intestines. In return for free food and a warm place to live, these gut bugs make medicines for you. (To meet your microbiome and learn about the medicines it makes, see our partner book, *The Dr. Sears T5 Wellness Plan*, and our book for children, *Dr. Poo.*)

4. **Your brain.** As the commander-in-chief of all the doctors, pharmacies, and medicines within your body, the brain communicates via biochemical text messages to the rest of your doctors within. (To learn more about the synergy between your brain and your other healing doctors within, see our partner book, *The Healthy Brain Book.*)

As you are growing your conquer-cancer mind, instead of dwelling on your fear, dwell on these doctors within, where they and their pharmacies are located, and how to open those pharmacies to dispense the right medicines for you. This mindset upgrade shifts your cerebral and physical energy into tools for healing—rather than wasting it fretting about "Why me?" "What did I do?" "What caused my cancer?"

To help that mindset shift, let's take a deeper dive in the next chapter into the first of these doctors within: your ISA.

I just got the diagnosis. How can I best share this news with my friends and loved ones? I need their support, but I don't want to freak them out.

Talk from your heart and your new conquer-cancer mindset. Try opening with, "I need to share with you some recent medical news and I need your support!" When they feel the positive vibes in your voice, they are more likely to join forces with their own uplifting replies, such as "We're praying for you!" and "You're such a wise person. We believe you will heal."

Remember, sad news is contagious. Your supporters are more likely to offer helpful advice if you have already shown a positive mindset.

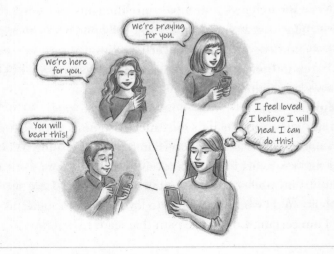

Testimonial: Lessons from a Doctor/Cancer Thriver

I was diagnosed with pancreatic cancer with metastasis to the liver on December 2, 2020.

As a naturopathic physician, I had lived the philosophy that I shared with my patients and the people in my life: I ate well, exercised, and supplemented my nutrition. In the months before my diagnosis, I actually felt (even within the context of COVID-19 changing my gym habits) that I was in great physical shape.

Then my world shifted, and with it, a new mindset emerged for me and those around me. When you have cancer, you become part of a family. I want that family to be one of love and not fear.

Cancer creates fear, and feelings of fear create an indelible change in your body's neurochemistry that none of us can afford. Fear also creates an energy in ourselves (and our community) that sends the wrong vibrational message to our cells regarding their healing.

Cancer is a part of our bodies; therefore, it is a part of our selves. How can you "fight" or "wage war" (all fear-based terminology, by the way) on your own body? It doesn't work. Like it or not, the cancer that is in you is a part of you—it came from you.

As I approach my cancer, there are thoughts and words that I use every day that are not fear-based. I call upon my healing powers. I acknowledge that my cancer is a message sent to educate me. I seek to understand that message and its origins. I believe that *my* cancer is partially the result of toxic emotions (especially resentment) that I have held in my body for too long.

I am a few months into my cancer diagnosis and treatment, and I am already whole-body certain that I am healing. With my mind and my heart filled with love, there is no room for fear or doubt. Of my ability to reach a state of remission, I am sure. Of my ability to do whatever it takes to love myself through this process, I am certain. Love is the path that leads to certainty.

So, how do we reframe the language of cancer from fear to love? For me, the answer to this question started immediately upon my diagnosis. Sitting with my oncologist, my nurse practitioner, and my nurse, I asked that we not discuss the "terminal" nature of my cancer nor the timelines related to my lifespan. For me, none of that information was relevant and acknowledging it by verbalizing it would trigger fearful feelings in me. "Terminal" is a frightening word and putting a timeline on your own death can be extremely terrifying. A terminal cancer diagnosis is a huge stressor, and stress impairs your immune system.

I tell myself that whatever I hear from my doctors (conventional or integrative) is just "information." Good test, bad test—it's just information. It informs and helps guide my decisions as I move forward in a proactive way. What I do with the information I receive, such as lab test numbers, is under my control.

Here's what I am doing, and it's working for me:

- I eat fresh, organic vegetables, fruit, and fish exclusively. No processed foods of any kind.
- I do not eat *any* sugar. Specifically, *no* added sugar.
- I eat a meal every two hours. I always have a snack available.
- I drink lots of spring or filtered water and sometimes I have tea. I love warm, unsweetened plant-based milks to which I add cinnamon and nutmeg as a treat.
- I exercise, which right now is walking and doing push-ups and sit-ups, as often as I can.
- I say a daily healing mantra and practice deep-breathing techniques.

From a treatment perspective, I have what I consider to be an exceptional team and an incredibly successful approach that includes the best of both conventional and integrative oncology.

The development of my integrative program took months to establish, and now that it is solidly in place, it is showing tremendously positive results on my overall wellness, strength, weight gain, and energy levels. My most recent CT scan results have shown that, since my December 2020 diagnosis, my pancreatic tumor has shrunk in two dimensions by 52 percent and my liver tumors are shrinking as well.

As I heal, I focus on the love of my family, the love of my life partner, and the passion I bring to my professional life. I am thankful for all of the support that I receive from everyone in my life. That positive joy boosts me and promotes the positive vibrational energy that I need.

I know, for myself, remaining positive comes down to the following:

- I don't stress.
- I do my best not to take on resentment.
- I understand and leverage the power of the information I receive about my cancer.
- I listen to my intuition.
- I live day to day and function proactively within my treatment program.
- In my mind, I have already moved past my cancer.

I offer these thoughts to you with all the love in my heart and wish you all the best.

Andrew Myers, ND, is a graduate of Bastyr University, Center for Natural Health, and has been a naturopathic physician for thirty years. He is the author of five books, including *Simple Health Value*, *Health Is Wealth*, *Health Is Wealth: Performance Nutrition for the Competitive Edge*, *The New Heart Health*, and, most recently, *Simplifying the COVID Puzzle*.

Chapter 2

. . . .

Meet Your Natural Conquer-Cancer Army Inside

If only there was a medicine that helped healthy cells get healthier and also helped keep cancer cells in check!

Good news: There is, and you make it inside your body. It's called your personal *immune system army* (ISA).

Like so many other ailments, cancer is an immune system imbalance.

> ### Cancer is an immune system imbalance.

As you read that, ponder how you start thinking differently. Just hearing the word "imbalance" (versus "disease") triggers thoughts of hopefulness and opens the door to having an action plan. Hope is healing. When we rightly see cancer as an immune system imbalance, it makes more sense that we can help heal it.

The word "immunity" stems from the Latin *immunitas,* meaning "freedom from." Let us extend the meaning to "freedom from cancer." A smarter immune system not only helps you conquer cancer but generally improves your quality of life.

Faith over fear. As part of your conquer-cancer mindset, dwell more on having faith in your immune system and less on your fear of cancer. (See the related section on spiritual faith over fear, page 147.)

Preload to prevent and heal. What you'll learn in this book will not just help you conquer the cancer you have. It will also show you how to "pre-load" your immune system for the future—equip your immune system army to fight smarter for you *before* it gets weak and you get sick.

Get ready to go inside your body to learn more about how cancer grows, and how your ISA fights it.

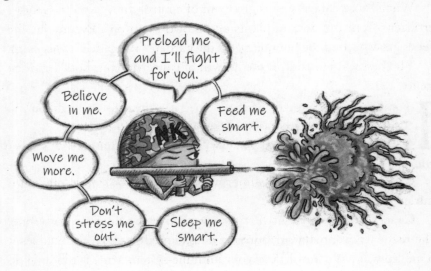

Why You Get Cancer: An Overview

Why did I get cancer? is often the first thought every person with cancer has. While it's unhelpful to dwell too much on what caused your cancer, it can be instructive to understand what's going on inside your body that shouldn't be. How did your immune system get out of balance?

Compare cancer to a garden growing out of control. Sometimes a genetic mix-up causes a healthy cell to become a cancer cell. Think of a cancer cell as a seed. How much and how fast this cancer "seed" multiplies depends on the soil around it. If the soil is fed cancer-fertilizing foods and pollutants, then the seed grows into a cancer plant, a dangerous weed that invades neighboring flowers and plants. Just as you want to keep your garden full of flowers and not weeds, you want the same in your body.

Your internal "soil" is your primary conquer-cancer tool. Consider the different rates of cancer in the United States versus Asia. People in Asia, especially the Japanese and Chinese, may carry as many microtumors as Westerners in their bodies, but they are less likely to become aggressive cancers because their soil (the typical Asian diet) is not as favorable to cancer growth as American soil (the standard American diet—SAD).

When those cancer weeds grow out of control, they steal nutrients— fertilizer—from the normal plants and crowd them out. Eventually, the weeds grow beyond the boundaries of the garden—the cancer *metastasizes*.

The best ways to control the growth of cancer in your body's garden are to:

- Keep the seeds from becoming cancerous, and
- Shut off their food and fertilizer so they can't grow.

Cancer specialists call this improving our *biological terrain*, making it unfriendly to cancer growth.

Cancer occurs mainly when two protective mechanisms go wrong. The tissue environment surrounding a "bad seed" cancer cell enables it to multiply out of control. And your immune-system army is too weak to search out and destroy the misbehaving cancer cell before it proliferates.

Every organ in your body is only as healthy as each cell in that organ. Cultivating healthy cells is sort of like raising a healthy child. The healthier the home and neighborhood environment, the healthier that child is likely to be. Yet, put a young cell in a toxic tissue environment, and the cell is more likely to misbehave and turn cancerous.

Leukemia is a good example of the cancer-garden analogy. Your bone marrow is your garden and your white blood cells (WBC) are one of its plants. When the soil, bone marrow, is "enriched" with cancer fertilizers (carcinogens), the healthy seeds and plants (WBC) "mutate" and become cancerous. The cancer cell then further misbehaves by making its own fertilizers; cancer cells produce vascular endothelial growth factor (VEGF) to feed their growth. VEGF is helpful when produced by normal cells, such as the lining of your blood vessels (see pages 130–131 on how your endothelium works). But inside a cancer cell, it stimulates more blood vessels to feed the cancer cell—what oncologists call *angiogenesis*. And if your immune-system army can't find and destroy the cell in time, it multiplies.

Which garden are you growing in your body?

> To prevent and heal from cancer:
> 1. Maintain a healthy cellular environment, and
> 2. Empower your natural immune-system
>   army to fight smarter for you.

A Second Helping of Why You Get Cancer: A Tale of Two Cells

Inside each cell is a genetic code that prompts the cell, "Increase and multiply, and when your job is over, 'retire' to make room for young, healthy cells to take your place." *Apoptosis*, the replacement of old cells with new cells, occurs trillions of times a day throughout your body. Yet sometimes the genetic signal gets garbled and keeps turning on the growth of a cell instead of turning it off. As a result, the cell becomes cancerous and multiplies out of control, and the cancer invades and damages surrounding tissue. Eventually, the process can creep into the bloodstream and travel throughout the body—a stage called *metastasis*.

Think of the conquer-cancer plan outlined in Part III of this book as first creating healthy cellular soil that prompts your genetic codes to keep

Apoptosis

A good cell that doesn't retire can turn into a cancer cell

cells healthy. Then, as a backup, it supports your immune system by recognizing cancer cells early enough to kill them before they have a chance to grow and spread.

A cancer cell is a selfish cell, focused on its own growth and survival, even at the expense of all of its buddy cells in the body. A friend of ours recently got breast cancer while still in her reproductive stage of life. Normally, the community of breast cells all work together to make milk, the function for which they were designed. But the selfish cancer cell inside the breast only cares about its own growth, even at the expense of wiping out all the milk-producing cells.

Cancer cells are also smart. Since their favorite grow-food is sugar (specifically, glucose), they maliciously morph their cell membranes into making more receptors, or doors that open to invite sugar to "Come on in!"

My genes made me get cancer! Usually not true. You may inherit a *tendency* toward getting cancer but not necessarily a "gene" for cancer. Most cancers are not inherited. In fact, over the past twenty years, "genetic predisposition" (that is, my parents had it, therefore, I might get it) has been downgraded to a minor cancer contributor. For example, the misbehaving genes *BRCA1* and *BRCA2* are considered contributors in only 5 percent of all breast cancers. Generally speaking, contributors to cancer are around 80 percent environmental and at the most 20 percent genetic.

This is good news! The emerging sciences *epigenetics* (how your lifestyle affects your genes) and *nutrigenetics* (how your eating habits influence your genes) are proving that the expression of our genetic tendencies is mostly under our control.

As you will learn on page 72, certain eating habits and lifestyles can cause cells to misbehave and multiply out of control, creating cancer. The four main factors that influence cell behavior are L.E.A.N.: lifestyle, exercise, attitude, and nutrition. Raise a cell in a healthy L.E.A.N. environment and you get less cancer.

In Part III you will learn how to use diet and lifestyle to put every cell in your body back into a healthy L.E.A.N. environment, to teach them to remain healthy, too.

Our soil becomes SAD. While we are not fans of numbers or statistics, one correlation stands out as reinforcing the idea that cancer occurs when we put the cells of our body into an environment they were not designed to be in. It just so happens that the rise of cancer in the United States has paralleled the changes in our lifestyle. Over the past fifty to seventy years, we began eating out of boxes rather than eating from farm to fork, a transition now called the standard American diet (SAD). We began to sit more and move less. We began to stress more. In a nutshell, we encouraged the seeds of cancer in our body by creating a soil environment that causes these cells to flourish.

Twin studies tell all. Identical twins tend to get the diseases of their adoptive families when they grow up, rather than those of their biological parents. Again, lifestyle is more cancer-contributing than genes.

Another scientific finding suggesting that the soil is more important than the seed was found when studying the indigenous societies of North America and Canada. People in these societies had a very low risk of cancer until the post–World War II food revolution of processed foods high in sugar and refined grains more than tripled their incidence of cancer. Similarly, women from cultures with a low incidence of certain cancers, such as the low breast cancer rates in Japan and China, had a two- to fourfold increase in risk when moving to the United States. In both cases, genes couldn't have changed that quickly. The difference had to be diet and lifestyle.

How good cells become bad. Genes produce (among many other things) enzymes, which are the internal language of cellular metabolism. They are what tell the cell to "grow, multiply, stay healthy, live long, do good things for the body." (Sounds like your mother!) Yet sometimes, biochemical intruders, called carcinogens, get into the cell and disrupt this healthy cellular communication. Carcinogens' bad language prompts the cell to grow and multiply out of control—to turn cancerous.

Realistically, with the challenges of living in a toxic world, we can't avoid all the carcinogens around us. We eat toxin-sprayed foods out of possibly carcinogenic containers, breathe toxic air, drink chemically treated water, and more. Yet we can *minimize carcinogens* as much as possible (see page 155), plus focus on *smartening our ISA* inside to better fight the cancer carcinogens. Let's start by taking a closer look at the immune system's role in fighting cancer.

Cancer Is a Body Out of Balance

Cancer is basically a body out of balance, beginning with the cells. Within our cells is a delicate balance of two sets of genes: cancer-promoting *oncogenes* (gas pedals) and tumor-suppressing *anti-oncogenes* (brake pedals). Normally, there is a balance between the two that is automatic. When this balance is disrupted in favor of the oncogenes—whether by carcinogens or diet and lifestyle, or even just by unlucky chance—you "get cancer."

Cancer healing, and future cancer prevention, means putting your body back in balance, starting with your immune system. Health in general is a balance of your immune system. We use the term "smarten" your immune system, but really, the best term is "balancing." You don't want to "strengthen" your immune system too much, or it can over-fight, or get confused, and start to kill healthy cells. This is what causes autoimmune illnesses. You want your immune system fighters to be selective and seek out germs and cancer cells and fight them, while leaving healthy tissues alone.

There are three big reasons you need to know your immune system army (ISA) inside:

1. Most cancers (like most diseases) stem from a weakened immune system.
2. Cancer itself can weaken your immune system, leaving you with an increased chance of getting other illnesses.
3. Changing your mindset to focus on your ISA rather than your cancer will help you heal.

Cancer hacks. Your immune system army continually patrols your body on the lookout for cancer cells. But cancer cells are sneaky and have a way of hacking the immune system. To survive, they either put the immune system to sleep, disabling its fighters, or put up a protective barrier, or disguise, so the immune system fighters don't recognize them as the bad guys. They're even able to entice some of your immune cells to become traitors by switching sides and joining the cancer cell army. Cancer cells can also "lie dormant," meaning they fly under the radar of your ISA. You may not feel them until they grow or spread years later.

The trillions of cells throughout our body are constantly multiplying, but some cells become cancerous when they multiply out of control. The sad news is we all have cancer cells in our bodies. The glad news is a healthy immune system kills these cells and stops cancer from growing.

Let's follow your top conquer-cancer army inside, a part of your immune system called *natural killer cells* (NK cells), to learn how they fight for you.

NK Cells: What They Are, What They Do, and How to Make Them Fight Better for You

NK cells remind me of my days making rounds as a doctor in the hospital. Our team's job was to be rapid responders, ready to rush to the scene to help with serious accidents or illnesses. That's what NK cells do. Your NK cells are the *rapid responders* that kill cancer cells.

Healthy noncancerous cells display a biochemical barcode (called MHC-1) that, in effect, tells the NK cell army, "Don't shoot—we belong

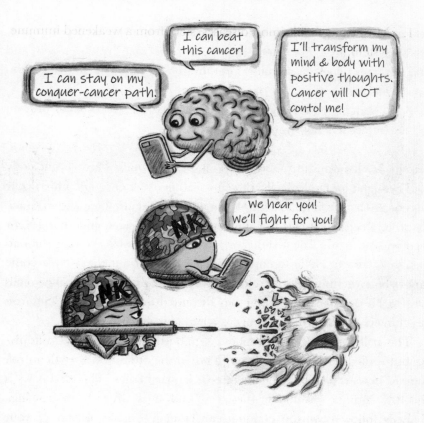

here!" When healthy cells turn cancerous, they lose their MHC barcode protection. Only if they manage to avoid the NK army's notice do they grow into a tumor.

Consider NK cells as the Navy Seals of your immune system. They are heavily armed, well-trained cellular soldiers that are constantly on a search-and-destroy mission. When an NK cell finds a cancer cell, it is magnetically drawn to it, and gloms onto it. It then uses biochemical bullets called *perforins* to literally poke holes into the cancer cell membrane and inject cancer cell–dissolving enzymes called *granzymes* into the cell to kill it. The defeated and deflated cancer cell then becomes cellular garbage, which is removed by macrophages ("big eaters"), your immune system's garbage collectors.

NK cells are called "natural" because, unlike other immune cells, they are programmed to pounce on virus-infected cells and cancer cells at first recognition. Other troops in your immune system army need prior expo-sure to be activated, the principle on which vaccines are developed, and what happens when you build up immunity to a flu virus only after pre-viously getting it.

NK cells originate in bone marrow and comprise 10 to 15 percent of the white blood cells in your bloodstream. Their job of protecting the "good guys" (healthy cells and tissues) and destroying the "bad guys" (can-cer cells) is accomplished using something called "receptors."

Throughout your body is a giant social network through which your cells communicate. The "messages" in this network are biochemical, usu-ally protein molecules that travel from sender to receiver, and are received by receptors—docks for the biochemical message ferryboats—on the mem-branes of cells. An NK cell sends a biochemical message that is "received" by the good guys, for which the bad guys don't have a receptor. The good guys send a text back that says, "I'm a friend. Don't bother me. Fight for me." If the NK cell detects the cell is a bad guy—it fights it.

The wiser, or healthier, the message and the smarter the NK cells, the more effective the communication. This is one of the main goals of our conquer-cancer plan to smarten your immune system.

Visualize your immune system team. Fascinating studies show that you can change how your immune system army fights for you with something called *guided imagery*, in which you visualize images of your cancer-fighting soldiers inside killing cancer cells and healing tissues. We know you can think-change your brain; you can also think-change your immune system, for better or worse. This is why positive people and optimists tend to have a healthier immune system than do negative people and pessimists.

Our conquer-cancer plan helps prevent and heal from cancer by two main mechanisms:

1. It provides a healthy soil around cells to keep them from turning cancerous, as you learned about on page 26.
2. It increases the number and fighting ability of your NK cells so you have a larger and better trained ISA inside.

That's cancer healing in a nutshell.

Five Ways to Help Your NK Cells Fight Smarter for You

If your NK cells could prompt you what to do (they do, but we often don't listen), they would offer these tips for how you should think, eat, move, sleep, and share:

1. "Believe in us; don't stress us out!"
2. "Feed us to fight better for you."
3. "Move more, sit less!"
4. "When you sleep better, we fight better."
5. "Help others heal. Share your healing plan."

Imagine holding these five keys to unlocking the potential of your NK cell army in the palm of your hand.

"Believe in Us; Don't Stress Us Out!"

Spend more thought time dwelling on "I trust my ISA to heal me" than on "I fear cancer." One of the most mysterious miracles in medicine is the observation that people with cancer who have a conquer-cancer mindset of self-empowerment have been shown to have smarter NK cells compared to patients who felt hopeless and helpless.

> Hope is healing.

Trusted immunologists theorize how this happens. When we believe we will heal, our body-mind sends a certain type of biochemical message, called cytokines (cell movers), to our NK cells that tells them: "We believe in you—now go fight those cancer cells."

Your NK cells are also sensitive to your emotions, which is why a happier and more hopeful mind results in more and smarter NK cells that are fiercer cancer fighters. NK cells have receptors that detect the level of circulating stress hormones, and they respond to these levels. They get weakened, or "stressed out," by stress hormone levels that stay high for too long.

In her must-read book, *Molecules of Emotion*, Dr. Candace Pert uncovers science supporting that people who are better in touch with their emotions (who are able to deal wisely with sad, happy, and angry thoughts) are more likely to have a smarter ISA and heal better from cancer.

How your emotions flow helps your ISA grow.

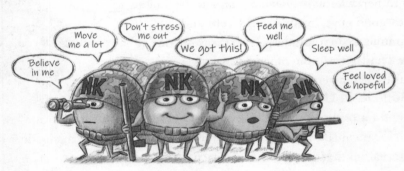

Help your natural conquer-cancer army
fight better.

Survivor Martha notes: *A study that affirmed my own belief effect was one where scientists at the National Cancer Institute studied two groups of women with breast cancer. Those who mastered their conquer-cancer mindset by dwelling on "I believe I will heal," "I feel empowered," and so on had a stronger cancer-fighting army of NK cells, healed better, and survived longer than did women who felt hopeless and helpless.*

Keep in Touch!

During her healing from breast cancer, Martha enjoyed getting backrubs, after which she seemed so relaxed. Bill's show-me-the-science curiosity clicked in. Sure enough, touch scientists have shown that women who enjoy several weekly massages while healing from breast cancer felt less stressed and showed increased NK cell activity.

Dwell on Dr. Bill's personal healing mantra: "I have cancer. I am not cancer!" Focus more on what you *can do* rather than what you *have*, and on the "good guys," your healthy cells and immune system inside. Hyperfocusing on the "bad guys," the cancer cells inside you, wastes healing energy.

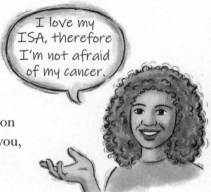

I love my ISA, therefore I'm not afraid of my cancer.

Name Your Conquer-Cancer Plan

Personalize your language to use the cancer-healing terms you prefer. We use terms like "fight" your cancer, and equip your immune-system "army." For some people, these military metaphors work and give them a sense of engagement. Others do not like the idea of a "war" within themselves and prefer to use language that reflects a focus on healing, health, and purpose.

Whatever you call the misbehaving cells inside, focus more attention on the *tools* you have rather than the rascal cancer cells. Although everyone is living with cancer cells inside, we must not let them control us.

"Feed Us to Fight Better for You."

As you will learn in Chapter 5, the smarter you feed your immune system army, the smarter it's likely to fight for you. Try to follow as many of the smart eight conquer-cancer diet tips as you can.

You will notice that our conquer-cancer diet section is the longest and most detailed in this book. That's because changing what and how you eat is likely to have the quickest and most lasting conquer-cancer (and prevent-cancer) effects.

"Move More, Sit Less!"

Movement mobilizes your immune system. Ponder the seven conquer-cancer medicinal effects of movement listed on page 126. There is no cancer drug in any pharmacy in the world that can match the cancer-healing and -preventing effects of exercise. Unlike prescription cancer drugs, the medicines you make when you move have only helpful and not harmful effects.

Exercise increases both the number and "killing" ability, called "cytolytic strength," of your NK cells. In a nutshell, movers have a higher number of NK cells and a smarter immune system army than do sitters. As an added perk, the increase in the number of NK cells you have is proportional to how smartly you exercise (see Chapter 6). If your NK cells could talk, they would say: "Move us more and we'll fight better for you!"

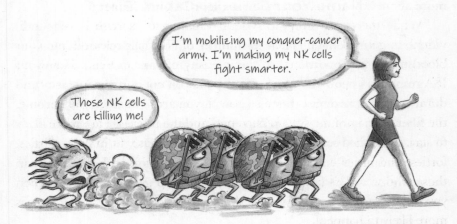

Movement mobilizes your conquer-cancer army.

Ready to go deeper? Imagine if you were in charge of strategy for your immune system army. Where would you station your NK cells so that they could be quickly mobilized? Answer: the lining of your blood vessels, called the *endothelium*. This allows your NK cells to quickly enter the bloodstream and travel anywhere in your body to attack germs and cancer cells.

Your white blood cells (WBCs)—your ISA troops, of which NK cells are just one type—take up camp in three areas of your body: your bloodstream, your tissues, and the lining of your blood vessels. In fact, only around 2 percent of your WBCs are actually in your blood. The rest are either in your tissues, doing their job, or ready and waiting, adhered to the lining of your blood vessels—called "marginated."

Around 50 percent of your WBC troops, including most of your NK cells, are stationed in the lining of your blood vessels. When you get up and exercise, the increased blood flow causes a "shear force" along that lining, prompting the NK cells to "demarginate," meaning separate from their resting place, increase their number in the bloodstream, and travel to a "homing destination" where they fight for you. Then, after exercise, many of these NK cells and other WBCs return to their endothelial camp.

Imagine taking a brisk walk with friends and boasting, "I'm mobilizing my natural immune system army inside." Or, if you really want to sound immune smart, "I'm demarginating my white blood cells." (See more about how movement mobilizes your ISA in Chapter 6.)

While the exact immune system response to exercise is very individual, in general the increase in number of NK cells released into your bloodstream is proportional to the intensity of your exercise. How your ISA responds to how you move also depends on not only the intensity and duration of your exercise, but also how fit you are. The fitter you become, the fitter your immune system becomes, and the fitter you are more likely to stay. Preloaded seniors—those who were previously fit in their thirties, forties, and fifties—usually enjoy better ISA function with exercise than those who were less fit. (This is a good reason to get off the couch when you're younger, to preload your ISA for when you're older and cancer is more likely to happen!)

Movement Mobilizes Your ISA

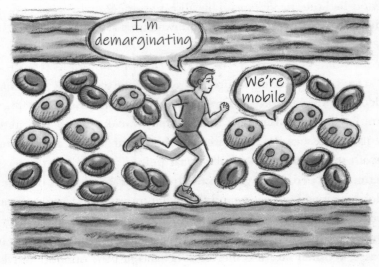

Sitting Stagnates Your ISA

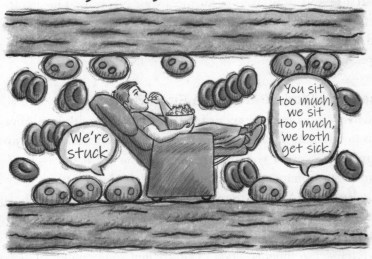

> ## View It and Do It!
>
> For a two-minute video clip on how movement opens your endo-thelial pharmacy, see youtube.com/watch?v=1fVzxsVJ7vA.

"What happens to our NK cell army when we get older?" you may be wondering. We are not convinced by the conclusion of some studies: that our immune system, like many other systems, weakens as a natural effect of aging. We believe the aging weakened immune system is more due to our *habits* than our age. Our take-home point is: the older you become, the more you need to move. Many sitters suffer from what doctors like Bill dub "the sitting disease" and also from immune system dysfunction. We believe there's a correlation. Another reason seniors need to sit less and move more: for many people, as they get older, their muscle mass decreases, yet their fat mass increases. This is just the opposite of what a smart ISA needs.

Go outside and play. Nature nurtures your NK cells. This makes sense since troops train out in the field. See why movement outdoors is smartly called "exercise squared" and how it smartens your ISA to fight better for you (page 135).

"When You Sleep Better, We Fight Better."

The correlation between sleep deprivation and cancer was discovered thanks to increases in cancer observed among habitual nightshift workers. During sleep is when your ISA reports for duty and starts cleaning up cellular messes, including cancer cells.

Consider this logic: Cancer happens when your ISA is imbalanced. Quality sleep improves ISA balance. Therefore, sleep better, fight cancer better.

NK cells love quality sleep. The greater your quality of sleep, the greater the quantity and quality of your NK cells. As an additional perk, a smarter nightshift ISA better targets germs. During cancer therapy and healing, many people suffer from more colds and other infections, known as "comorbidities."

Sleep deprivation has a double fault: you weaken your ISA, especially NK cells, but you also produce biochemical changes that feed cancer cells.

For more information about the sleep–cancer connection, see Chapter 8.

"Help Others Heal. Share Your Healing Plan."

Since your immune system is so sensitive to your emotions, engaging with and helping friends helps you feel better about yourself. As you are learning the language of cancer healing, formulating your personal healing plan, and journaling your journey, share your experience with others healing from cancer, especially those who have been recently diagnosed.

Imagine this dialogue between you and a friend:

"I can't stop thinking about my cancer," your friend confesses. "What do you think about during the day?"

"I dwell on my ISA, my immune system army inside. I remind myself what I can do to keep my ISA fighting better for me."

"Wow, tell me more about this ISA. That sounds like what I need to do!"

Then you download. As you are sharing and teaching what you have learned, you will be amazed at how natural it feels to explain the complex and confusing topic of your ISA in riveting, easy-to-understand terms.

Dr. Bill notes: *Over my fifty years as a doctor and voluntary professor, I have treasured the double effect you get when you share what you have learned: you learn it better and you feel good about sharing it, a feeling I call the "helper's high."*

Make Your Own Immunotherapy

Immunotherapy refers to using drugs to prompt a person's own ISA, especially the NK cells, to fight smarter. While researching this exciting new field of cancer therapy, Dr. Bill realized: "Hey, that's what our book is all about—making your own immunotherapy medicines!"

Part II

How to Wisely Partner with Your Cancer-Care Providers

A better prepared patient is a wiser partner. Now that you're in the right frame of mind for the many wise decisions you will now need to make—now that "I can conquer my cancer!" is your new normal—it's time to learn how best to work with the team of experts who will be helping you conquer your cancer.

Chapter 3

. . . .

What to Expect from Your Cancer- Treatment Team: An Overview

A s soon as you get the diagnosis "You've got cancer!" your first thought may be, "What happens now?" Now you meet the team of medical experts who will help you heal.

The first team member you are likely to meet is your *oncologist*, your conquer-cancer team quarterback, who will advise you on what other specialties you are likely to need and recommend specific team members to meet those needs. Your oncologist will discuss with you what surgery you need, if any, and may also discuss if you need cancer-healing prescription medicines (chemotherapy) and/or targeted X-ray treatments (radiation therapy).

Next, expect to meet one or more specialists in cancer surgery. If your oncologist believes you need surgery, your surgeon will discuss with you what's involved with the surgery, what to expect from your hospital, a general description of what type of surgery they will do, and how it's designed to help you. (See tips on how to wisely work with your surgeon on page 70.)

After surgery, you'll meet with your oncologist again to discuss the details of your chemotherapy, if needed: at what dose, for how long, and so on. Your oncologist will explain how the chemotherapy is designed to treat your particular cancer, what adverse effects you may feel, and how the research shows the chemotherapy helps conquer your cancer.

Your meeting with a *radiation oncologist*, if necessary, to discuss types of radiation therapy, how many treatments, and what adverse effects may occur, usually comes after meeting with your oncologist and surgeon. Yet, with some cancers, radiation is performed before either the surgery or chemotherapy. This is part of the plan that will be discussed with you on your first visit with your oncologist.

Other team members that may be available to you, especially in cancer centers affiliated with the National Cancer Institute, are a personal certified cancer coach, a cancer nutritionist, and other therapists whose specialties help you heal better and feel better. Oncologists are fond of explaining cancer as weeds in a garden. Surgeons, conventional oncologists, and radiation oncologists are the weed-pullers and killers. As the weeds are being pulled and killed, the rest of your healing team teaches you about and supports you on fertilizing the soil in your body's garden, to keep healthy plants (your cells) growing while not letting the weeds get out of control.

Become a Certified Health Coach

To help make cancer-healing your hobby, become a Dr. Sears Wellness Institute certified health coach. Our online courses not only help you heal, but also give you the tools to help others heal. You will be amazed when during a coaching session with a client you discover yourself advising something brilliant and feeling, "Oh, that advice just came out of me instinctively. That was good! I'm going to use that to help myself heal, too." (To find out how to get certified, see DrSearsWellnessInstitute.org.)

Cancer Speak: Terms You Must Know

During your journey to healing you will need to learn a new language. When you meet your team, it's helpful to already know the language they speak. The following are terms you will hear, read, and speak:

Cancer. From the Greek word *karkinos,* meaning "crab," because under a microscope, the extra blood vessels that protrude from cancer cells appear to drape over the tumor like crab feet.

Apoptosis. From a Greek word meaning "falling off." Imagine all cells being stamped with an expiration date that says when their job is over and they can retire; that's their apoptosis. Normal cells obey their expiration date; cancer cells ignore this date and keep on growing and invading.

Oncology. From a Greek word meaning "swelling," since tumors present as swellings. Oncology is the medical specialty dealing with cancer science and cancer treatment.

Surgery. A procedure that physically removes a cancer tumor, or as much of it as possible, by cutting into the body, while being careful to avoid affecting normal adjacent tissue.

Chemotherapy. The use of highly researched drugs designed to kill cancer cells via IV or pill. You may receive multiple drugs during chemotherapy. The rationale behind this is similar to using more than one antibiotic to kill an infection. Ideally, and somewhat theoretically, more drugs kill more of the cancer cells and leave fewer cancer cells behind to develop resistance to these drugs. That is the golden wish of cancer treatment: to kill 100 percent of the cancer cells and leave none to regrow.

Radiation therapy. The use of targeted X-ray beams to kill cancer cells.

Survival rate. What percentage of people with your type and stage tend to survive and for how long. But remember, everyone's cancer, and everyone's cancer-fighting ability, is unique. We suggest you not pay attention to these percentages until first discussing them with your oncologist. (For a deeper understanding of survival rate, see page 57.)

Personalized cancer treatment. Also called "integrative cancer therapy," this approach to cancer treatment takes into account a person's own individual L.E.A.N. habits, age, stage, blood tests, and other factors that help the doctor arrive at a customized treatment plan.

Complementary and alternative medicine (CAM). A medical product or practice that is used together with (complementary) or instead of (alternative) standard medical care. Usually, less is known about most types of CAM than about standard treatments, which go through a long and careful research process to prove they are safe and effective. CAM may include dietary supplements, megadose vitamins, herbal preparations, special teas, acupuncture, massage therapy, magnet therapy, spiritual healing, and meditation. (See Chapter 4 for how to blend CAM and traditional cancer treatments into the personalized treatment plan that is right for you.)

"Progression-free survival." This is the sweet phrase you want to hear from your oncologist. It means that not only have you survived the cancer, but it's somewhat unlikely to return. This is the dream of every patient and oncologist.

For a deeper discussion of the cancer terms you need to know, check out the *National Cancer Institute Dictionary of Cancer Terms* at cancer.gov/publications/dictionaries/cancer-terms.

How to Talk to Your Child About Their Cancer

If you're reading this book not because you have cancer, but because your child does, you may be wondering: How do you talk to them about their cancer in a way that gives them a conquer-cancer mindset and sets them up to be a good partner in their cancer healing?

Parenting, in a nutshell, is teaching your children *tools to succeed in life*. Give them their own conquer-cancer tool kit.

Start by personalizing your dialogue to fit your child's age and medical needs:

"Your beautiful body is made up of lots of tiny cells. These cells are constantly growing and multiplying. That's how you grow so big and beautiful. Sometimes these nice cells become *naughty* cells. They grow too big, too fast. They invade some organs and sometimes they try to hurt your nice cells. The battle begins. But, don't worry, dear. God put inside your strong body a big army to eat up those naughty cells to keep them from hurting your nice cells. Let's look inside your body and see how your army fights for you."

Then play show-and-tell about NK cells from pages 30–32. Even better, use these illustrations as a guide to draw your own that fit your child's level of understanding.

During your dialogue, expect to need to excuse yourself. Say "I have to go potty," then retreat for a few minutes to have a good cry, put aside your distress, and take a deep breath. Afterward, put on your best smile and return to teaching your child tools for healing *and for life*.

"You are blessed with a team of healers: your doctors and your parents. Your doctors will give you medicines to get rid of those naughty cells. We will teach you what you can do—self-help skills to help your smart army of NK cells fight those naughty cells and grow more nice cells."

Remember, just as kids like to nibble on food, they also like small, frequent helpings of healing tips. Periodically stop and listen to your child repeat to you what they are processing from the tools you are teaching.

Finally, share with your child our mantra for all ages: Dwell more on your *conquer-cancer army inside* than the cancer in you.

And if you want more help: Inquire if your child's hospital has a cancer-healing support network that you can join. Visit childrensmiraclenetwork.org for more resources.

Get Your Cancer "Vaccine"

"What! I didn't know there was a cancer vaccine," you may be thinking. That depends on your definition of "vaccine." The CDC definition is "a product that stimulates a person's immune system to produce immunity to a specific disease." Consider the usual childhood vaccines that have so greatly lessened those dreadful diseases like smallpox and polio. You get a shot, such as a polio vaccine, that teaches the body to make antibodies (anti-polio fighters) against the disease so you don't get it.

Regarding cancer, we like to think of a "vaccine" as anything you can take, make, or do that prompts your body's own immune system to help you prevent getting cancer and help you heal from cancer. Consider the tools you will learn—and use—as being like making your own vaccine against most types of cancers. Unlike the usual vaccines that simply require one or more shots and an occasional "booster" shot to keep those antibodies up, your personalized vaccine requires small, daily (even hourly) "doses" over a long period of time—perhaps even a lifetime of "daily boosters." But when you take this "vaccine" on schedule (the earlier in life you start, the better it works) and in the right doses for your body, it may prevent cancer, lessen the severity of cancer, and help you heal.

Our definition aside, you may be pleasantly surprised to also learn that the National Cancer Institute has a branch called the Laboratory of Tumor Immunology and Biology (LTIB), whose aim is to develop a cancer vaccine that smartens the immune system to target tumors. Your oncologist may discuss with you some recent "targeted therapies" that fit your individual cancer (see page 67). In the meantime, do the tools in our conquer-cancer plan and MYOCV—*make your own cancer vaccine.*

Chapter 4

. . . .

Partnering with Your Cancer-Care Providers

When wise patients partner with wise cancer-care providers, they bring out the best in each other. In this chapter you will learn how to talk so your cancer-care providers will listen, and listen so your cancer-care providers will talk. We'll teach you the tools we've seen people with cancer find most helpful, and the ones cancer-care doctors want their patients to use.

Prepare Yourself for Your First Consultation

When you first meet with your oncologists about your cancer treatment plan, you are probably still working through your "You've got cancer!" shock, and that can affect your ability to find your personal path to healing. Most newly diagnosed people are "stressed out" of thinking clearly. The better you prepare, the less you worry.

During your early meetings with your cancer doctors, not only are you seeking solid information, so are they. Cancer specialists are trained to discern whether you are very scared or well prepared. Imagine your oncologist asking, "How are you feeling?" You quickly respond, "Doctor, I'm prepared. I'm reading this book, *Help Heal Yourself from Cancer*. I'm not wasting mental energy on fear, and I'm putting together my personal plan to conquer my cancer." You have just set the stage for getting the best from your oncologists.

Oncologists think: *On the first visit, my patients are often so overwhelmed that they don't process half of what I'm saying.*

Get screen smart. Naturally, within minutes of getting your diagnosis, you'll want to reach for the keyboard to see what "Dr. Search Bar" says. Don't! You will be overwhelmed with information at the very time your mind is least prepared to be selective about what is the right information for you.

Mind first, information second. Before you let in lots of statistics and hundreds of "do this" and "take this" opinions, read and ponder our section on developing your conquer-cancer mind in Part I. Remember, you are "vulnerable" to both well-meaning friends and money-hungry internet promotions. Program yourself to be wise and selective about what you read and hear. This is your cancer, and your mindset is the starting line on your path to healing. Keep your mind uncluttered.

Read up! Two weeks before your first appointment with your cancer-care provider (or as soon as possible, if your appointment is less than two weeks away), send the office an email with this request: "Doctor, please send me your top, most-trusted articles, books, and online resources that I can look at to be better prepared for our upcoming appointment." The more familiar you become with your cancer, the less anxious you will feel—and the more personalized the cancer treatment you are likely to get. Also, by requesting this from your doctor and not a search engine, you make sure the information you get is science-based. You are asking your doctor to help you be more selective with your homework.

Or, if you are already in consultation with your cancer-care provider, at your next appointment try: "Doctor, will you please email me your three top articles and recommended resources for me to read for my type and stage of cancer? And please highlight sections of the resources that most fit my individual cancer and the points you want me to consider."

Oncologists advise: *The main mistake newly diagnosed cancer patients make is they get too much advice too soon, much of which is not specific for their cancer. Instead, they should ask their trusted oncologist to select the most scientific articles that most closely match their cancer and their general health.*

Preload your oncologist. A few days before each appointment, email your oncologist a one-page, bullet-point, at-a-glance overview of what you are feeling, reading, and doing. Here's an example for your first appointment:

- I'm gradually becoming more hopeful and less fearful.
- I'm reading *Help Heal Yourself from Cancer.*
- Could we please omit scary statistics and words like "survival percentages" and "terminal" unless you believe those stats will lessen my fear.
- I'm on the fence about . . . but I trust your expert advice. (See why we recommend this phrasing, page 60.)

Be Wise and Open-Minded

Notice we say "wise," not "smart." "Wise" upgrades "smart," meaning how you apply what you learn to the cancer you have.

Be selectively open-minded. If you are feeling "I want to try everything," share this dilemma with your doctor, who can then help filter the many pieces of advice you read and hear. After, focus on which ones seem right for you.

Consult a cancer-research specialist. After your oncologist provides you with selected resources, it's likely you will need professional guidance and a crash course in how to wisely read scientific articles. Try these steps:

1. Ask your oncologist to interpret the top points of each article that most pertain to *you*.
2. Ask, "Doctor, how would you rate this article?"
3. Seek a second opinion (see also page 66). Contact a cancer center in your state or region designated by the National Cancer Institute and ask for a second opinion. This could be an in-person visit or a virtual encounter, and might include recommendations about a treatment plan and/or sources of additional information.

To chemo or not to chemo? That is the question. "I'm not going to get that awful chemo!" is what some people may think. Others may think, "Just give me everything to kill my cancer." Better is to think, "I really need to be sure I need chemo, and what type of chemo." Approaching such a decision with an emphatic "I'm not going to get chemo!" may block your mind from formulating the right treatment plan for you.

Whatever the treatment prescribed for your cancer, it's wise to:

- Ask to see supportive science that fits your type and stage of cancer, your age, and your general level of health, to create a personalized plan (see page 58).
- Seek further opinions and expert help on interpreting the research (see above).
- Ask about "the tipping point" (see pages 62–64).

Ask for a Personalized Plan

Personalized cancer treatment, also called "integrative cancer therapy," takes into account a person's own individual L.E.A.N. habits, age, stage, blood tests, and other factors to help the doctor arrive at a customized treatment plan.

You Are a Person, Not a Percentage

Oncologists are "numbers doctors." They need to be. Cancer treatment protocols—the "standards of care"—are based on *statistics*: a patient with this type and stage of cancer, receiving these treatments, has this chance of survival. And that "survival rate" is based on the outcomes of a large number of people with a certain type of cancer receiving certain types of treatment. For example, a study that compares a chemo pill with a placebo pill might find "people taking this chemo enjoyed a survival rate at five years that is 10 percent greater than matched controls taking a placebo."

However, *you are a person, not a number.* You will read and hear statistics such as "patients with your cancer have a __ percent chance of healing from it," and so on. But it would be nearly impossible to categorize a few thousand people with the same cancer according to their age, stage, associated health conditions, level of leanness, conquer-cancer mindset, support resources, level of conquer-cancer diet, and so on. This is why some statistical studies may be a misfit for you.

Question the survival rate. While the survival rate for your cancer and treatment is important, don't take it "personally." Each person's cancer cells and each person's ability to fight cancer is unique. Many of the older studies don't take this into consideration. Fortunately, newer studies are trying to correct this defect by using people with your age, stage, and L.E.A.N. habits to arrive at a more accurate percentage—a "personalized survival rate." This is very challenging for cancer researchers to do, but it's better for you.

Keep in mind, also: You deserve both quantity and *quality* of life. When deciding on type and length of treatment, survival rate is vital, but so is your quality of life, which can be very difficult for cancer studies to measure. Yes, you want to "survive" longer, but you also want to thrive longer. One of the biggest challenges for oncologists is prescribing a treatment plan that targets a longer life while also causing a minimum of adverse reactions. (See "tipping point," pages 62–64.)

Want to shine as a savvy patient? Ask about cohort studies. "Cohort" is research-speak for a group of people whose age and stage of cancer and general level of health closely match your own. Realistically, there are no perfect cancer cohorts. Everyone's cancer is unique and so is the fighting ability of each person's immune system. But cohort studies are still better than generic survival rates.

At present, cohort studies are the weakest point in the $5 billion a year spent on cancer research. The best cohort studies would include at least a thousand people with your type and stage of cancer, your age and general health, and your L.E.A.N. habits. Be prepared for an answer such as, "We don't have cohort studies that exactly match what you are asking."

Push for a personalized answer. "Doctor, since I am lean, healthy, and have a smart immune system, do you believe I could qualify for a safer schedule of treatments?" Perhaps a certain chemo dose and length of treatment is recommended, yet you happen to be a person with a positive conquer-cancer mind who is lean and a "health nut," with a smart immune system. You may warrant more or less treatment than the standard of care suggests. The drug and the dose need to be personalized to treat *you*. (See Martha's personalized treatment story, page 60, and Dr. Bill's similar stories, pages 63 and 67.)

The Oncologist's Dilemma

Trusted oncologists certainly have the best interest of their patients in mind, yet many feel somewhat limited by two factors: the standard of care, and the lack of scientific studies on other patients that fit the age, stage, and general health of each unique patient.

Oncologists often feel obligated to follow the standard of care (which, most of the time, is based solely on survival rate, a statistic we know does not take an individual's cancer-fighting ability into account). Imagine your oncologist's challenge: When they follow a standard protocol, at least they know it works for many patients. Asking them to personalize a protocol just for you may feel "riskier" to them than relying on standard recommendations about which medicine, which dose, for what length of time, and so on.

Dr. Bill "gets personal." *When Martha was diagnosed with breast cancer, she fortunately had the benefit of personalized therapy—because, thanks to our previous experience with my colon cancers, we knew to ask for it. This was somewhat challenging for the oncologist, though, because it's easier and sometimes more mainstream to simply go with the statistics or "standard of care."*

Ask and you shall receive. The more you insist on a personalized cancer treatment plan, the more likely you are to get it. If you ask to work with your team of cancer-care providers to personalize your treatment, they are likely to oblige, which could reward you with not only a longer life but higher quality of life, too.

A comforting reply one of our trusted oncologists frequently inserted while listening to our questions was, "I hear you!" Your doctor should take your request seriously, and if they disagree, take the time to explain why.

How Insisting on a Personalized Treatment Plan Spared Martha Chemotherapy

After Martha had her expert surgery for breast cancer and recovered well, she was then on track toward chemo. Chemo kills cancer cells, but also at the expense of weakening much of the rest of your body. It can be lifesaving, but both the type of drug and duration of treatment need to be carefully selected to fit each person's individual cancer.

When Martha's oncologist asked how we felt about getting chemo, we answered, "We're on the fence." During that appointment to explain and schedule Martha for chemo, we presented a list of questions we wanted her doctor to ponder and answer to not only select the best chemo but also to be sure she needed it. We asked the oncologist to consider "personalizing" her treatment plan. Martha wanted more than just the statistics.

In particular, we wanted a sample of the tumor that was removed during her surgery to be given the Oncotype DX test. This breakthrough in genetic (read: personalized) testing predicts how likely your tumor is to respond to chemotherapy and helps guide your oncologist in selecting your treatment. This test grades the tumor tissue on a scale of 1 to 100, where the lower the number is, the less likely you are to need chemo. Her oncologist agreed to do this test, saying, "I would be pleasantly surprised if it teaches us anything." A week later we got a call from our trusted oncologist, who confided, "Martha, I must admit I am pleasantly surprised. Your score is 11. Based on this, chemo will not help. You don't need chemo."

Had we not asked the right questions and motivated her doctor to upgrade her treatment plan to include testing her individual tumor biology in his search for the right answers, Martha may have gone on to unnecessarily suffer the debilitating effects of chemo. (For more information on oncotyping, see oncotypeiq.com.)

Dr. Bill advises: *During my fifty years as a doctor, I have grown to value patients who upgrade themselves to being a "partner." When they challenge me to provide solid science, it keeps me motivated to pay particular attention to recent advances and provide them with the best science and care. In a nutshell, the more prepared and educated the "partner," the better care they are likely to get from the provider.*

Discuss Adverse Effects and the Concept of the Risk/Benefit Ratio

Two terms you are likely to hear from your cancer-care providers are "side effects" and "adverse effects," and you must know the difference. "Side effects" are mild discomforts that accompany many drugs, such as nausea, fatigue, and so on—aches and pains that are common, yet seldom interfere with your quality of life and usually quickly subside when treatment ends.

"Adverse effects," in contrast, interfere with your quality of life enough for your oncologist to stop the drug or lower the dose. For example, mild bone pain is a side effect; bone loss is an adverse effect. Be accurate and honest about how the drugs being used to treat your cancer are affecting your quality of life. "Doctor, I just can't go on like this . . ." merits a wise change in treatment.

We recommend asking your doctor early: "What adverse effects can I expect from my treatment, and is there anything I can start doing now to lessen these effects?"

Your doctor may respond with something like this: "You just asked about the number-one challenge that all doctors have, but especially oncologists. All the treatments we prescribe, in particular chemotherapy and radiation therapy, come with a risk/benefit ratio. Our goal is to prescribe a treatment regimen that gives you the highest benefits of healing with the lowest risk of painful reactions.

"The challenge is that, just as no two cancer cells and no two patients are alike, neither are their occurrence of adverse reactions. *Individual* and *not totally predictable* sums up our challenge. All we have are studies that show averages—it's those numbers again.

"I can tell you ahead of time what you might expect, such as fatigue, pain, nausea, intestinal upsets, brain fog, and so on, yet we won't know what you'll experience until we start the treatment. This is why both you and I need to prepare ourselves to be flexible, in case midway through your treatment you suffer more adverse effects, the risk/benefit ratio becomes high, and we need to modify our treatment plan."

By asking your cancer-care provider about the concept of adverse effects, you're increasing your chances of getting a treatment plan that is both effective in helping you heal from cancer and safe for your body. You want to heal from cancer, but you also want to minimize how sick you will be while you're healing.

Confide in your doctor. If you are worried about a proposed treatment or are experiencing painful adverse effects of treatment, say so! Your doctor relies on your feedback. Hiding it harms both you and your treatment plan.

During our follow-up visit with her radiation oncologist, when Martha downplayed the pain she was suffering from her radiation treatment for breast cancer (see page 64), her "scribe," Bill, stepped in and told her doctor how intense it seemed to be for her. Seeing the look of love and concern on Bill's face, her doctor immediately agreed to pause her treatment, allowing her to have a one-week break.

Research Your "Tipping Point"

During our cancers, we realized that there was a missing ingredient in the overall recommendations for chemotherapy and radiation therapy dosage, selection, and length of treatment. We call this the "tipping point." In each form of cancer treatment, you reach a point at which, while your survival rate may go up a few percentage points if you continue with the treatment, adverse effects skyrocket. That's when it may be wise to cut off treatment.

Determining your personal tipping point will be one of the most difficult decisions that you and your oncologist partner will need to make, mainly because it has not been researched like survival rate. The tipping point is not commonly considered in cancer treatment plans, presently, because it necessarily varies from patient to patient and has not been well researched. And you may not know your personal tipping point until you start to feel it ("After twenty treatments, my chest hurt so much I had to pause my treatment").

Play show-and-tell. You may wish to show your oncologist your understanding of the "tipping point." Be prepared to explain your concern in terms such as, "Doctor, if you recommend that I do chemo and/or radiation therapy, how many doses will I need?" Say the doctor recommends thirty doses. You then go deeper: "Doctor, in your experience and according to the science, at what dose is the 'tipping point,' when the dosage helps only a little but harms quality of life a lot?" Be prepared for an answer like, "We don't know. We do know that the thirty-dose protocol provides the usual survival percentage of 70 percent. We don't know what the survival rate of twenty doses is."

Dr. Bill's tipping point story. *The year was 1997. I had just recovered from expert surgery for colorectal cancer, and after surgery came chemo. I required intravenous chemotherapy instead of just popping a daily pill, and so for a few weeks, during my extended lunch hour while working at Sears Family Pediatrics, I went to get my intravenous chemo. So far, so good. Then came my daily trips to lie under an X-ray machine to get the area radiated. At the time, radiation therapy was so confusing that even medical doctors like me had a hard time understanding it. So, I just went along with my trusted radiation oncologist.*

Around 90 percent of the way through my radiation treatment, I was having such debilitating side effects that one night I had an aha! moment. I had reached a "tipping point," at which the slight increase in survival rate from continuing my radiation therapy paled in comparison with the probability of a huge increase in tissue damage and long-term serious side effects. I remember the next day discussing my "tipping point" concept with my trusted radiation oncologist. I told her I had decided to stop my radiation therapy and not continue with the 20 percent more as prescribed.

Several weeks later at a medical gathering, when I was pretty much back to feeling normal, I remember her consoling words to me: "You made the right decision to stop your treatment when you did. I just could not prescribe that dosage because it is below the standard of care."

Tame Your Treatment Anxiety

Nearly every person with cancer, and to a lesser extent their cancer-care providers, suffers from varying degrees of concern about their treatment: "If I don't treat my cancer aggressively enough, will it be more likely to return? Yet if I treat it too aggressively, am I likely to spend the rest of my life as a survivor but not a thriver, suffering with adverse effects?"

Martha shares: *Both Bill and I experienced high doses of treatment anxiety during my radiation therapy for breast cancer. While all three of us (Bill, myself, and my oncologist) were at peace that I didn't need chemo thanks to our research into cancer-cell aggressiveness (see page 60), the radiation therapy science seemed somewhat nebulous. Looking back, Bill and I wondered if my tipping point could have been twenty-three treatments, the point at which I was suffering so much from the radiation burn to my skin that I had to take a break. Yet, since the "standard of care" was twenty-eight treatments, I agreed to getting the full twenty-eight treatments (after taking a week off to recoup somewhat), plus five more lower-energy "boost" treatments, because I was anxious that I might have regrets years down the road about not listening to my oncologist and instead choosing to stop his prescribed treatments early.*

Dr. Bill shares: *Being married to this precious person for fifty-five years, when she hurts, I hurt. While we were blessed with excellent surgical and oncology care, I also suffered a dose of treatment anxiety. My doctor's mind perceived radiation therapy science as the least convincing in the whole field of cancer treatment. The "boost" recommendation of five extra doses was based on weak science—strike one! The possible increase in survival rate from the "boost" was only around 2 percent—strike two! Some noted oncologists even expressed concern that, in 1 percent of women, getting the "boost" could trigger a cancer in that radiated area (at the incision line only)— strike three! Also, there were no cohort studies of radiation therapy for her particular age, stage, and general level of health to help inform our decision. Our treatment anxieties prevailed and Martha committed to the full thirty-three treatments. Her* *doctor explained that the "boost" was a different type of radiation beam, at a much lower energy, specific to the incision line, and, trusting the doctor's judgment, we went ahead as recommended.*

Dr. Bill's Treatment Anxiety Advice to a Patient

One of my closest friends, let's call him Jack, called me recently, and I felt the anxiety in his voice as he shared, "Bill, my dear wife just had surgery for very early-stage lung cancer and now she's refusing chemo and radiation therapy. Please talk with her."

Here's my conversation with Jill:

"Jill, tell me about your decision about whether or not to have chemo and radiation therapy."

(I wanted to hear her reasoning since she is a wise person with a PhD in psychotherapy.)

"I don't want either. I'm refusing both," she said emphatically.

Immediately I put on three hats: cancer-healer, doctor, and self-trained psychotherapist (happily married for fifty-five years).

"Tell me about how you arrived at your decision," I responded *nonjudgmentally.*

"I've heard about those horrible side effects, and I don't want them!" she shared.

"What are you going to say to your oncologist?" I asked.

"'Doctor, I don't want either chemo or radiation therapy,'" she replied.

"Jill," I explained, "realistically, you can't and shouldn't make that decision on your own. Stating your belief in that way to your oncologist is a double fault." (Jill plays tennis.) "First, it sets you up for a severe case of treatment anxiety should your cancer come back. Second, it could put your oncologist off wanting you as a patient.

"Please try this approach instead: As soon as your doctor gives you an opener, such as 'Jill, how do you feel about beginning

---

chemotherapy and radiation therapy?' answer, 'Doctor, *I'm on the fence*. While I'm leaning toward not getting one or both, *I trust your advice*. It would help my decision anxiety if you could send me your three most trusted articles on both chemo and radiation therapy that address my concerns, including cohort studies or research on chemo and radiation therapy for my type of cancer, my age and stage, my general health, and my immune system health. It would also be helpful if you would highlight the percent survival rate in the treatment versus nontreatment groups, the percent risk of adverse effects, and the dosage that addresses my concern about the 'tipping point.'"

This type of dialogue works and *it's best for you*. First, you set your oncologist up to actually make the final decision, not you. Otherwise, you are setting yourself up for the blame game of "I should have been more open-minded," and so on, in case your cancer returns or progresses.

Second, your response instantly gets your cancer-care provider's attention, prompting them to think, "This is a sharp patient." Instead of falling back on "Well, it's the standard of care," they must personalize your treatment, including what treatment to get, what dose, and so on. It also motivates your oncologist to seek updated research and other opinions on chemo and radiation therapies for your particular cancer.

Seek Second Opinions and Sometimes Third and Fourth Ones

Among all the fields of medicine, cancer care is the one that still most suffers from diverse opinions and has not produced an increased level of care consistent with the huge number of research dollars it receives. If you need a second opinion, we recommend getting it from a National Cancer Institute–designated cancer center.

Dr. Bill's chemo-selecting story. *After my leukemia diagnosis, I started my cancer-care provider selection task. I needed chemo and wanted to take advantage of one of the greatest scientific breakthroughs in chemotherapy in cancer history, targeted therapy. The first oncologist I consulted wanted to put me on the strongest drug available. That didn't feel right because of the tipping point concept I had learned from my previous cancer, where the trade-off for survival rate going up slightly was morbidity rate going up hugely. The stronger the drug, the stronger the side effects. The second oncologist I spoke to wanted to put me on a newer form of targeted therapy, yet it had similar adverse effects.*

Then I realized I could get a third opinion from an oncologist who actually participated in some of the original treatment trials of this type of chemotherapy. My search led me to Dr. Richard Van Etten, director of the UCI Cancer Center, who looked at my whole profile and sent me some articles that he had authored on studying this therapy. Unlike the first two oncologists, he thought the best fit for me would be to start with the drug that had the longest track record and the least adverse effects. In other words, he wanted to go with the philosophy of "start low and go slow" rather than "hit hard and hope." The rest is my healthful cancer-healing history. At this writing, my chronic myelogenous leukemia is 99.99 percent undetectable. Thank you, Dr. Van Etten!

Share your concern. Be sure to confide in your primary oncologist that you are seeking other opinions and particularly if you seek other avenues of therapy. Suppose you decide to go with conventional therapy and a conventional oncologist. Yet you also seek consultation with an integrative oncologist (an oncologist who specializes in personalized treatment plans), to get the best of both worlds. By communicating that you are working with both, you are conveying to all of your cancer-care providers that you want the best blend of both, and when it comes to cancer therapy, you're more likely to get the level of care that you are seeking.

Should You Add an Integrative Oncologist to Your Team?

Conventional and integrative oncology can balance one another. For example, the radiation or chemo treatment recommended by your conventional oncologist may have a very high risk/benefit ratio, where your survival rate may go up a few percentage points while your morbidity rate goes up a lot more. Your integrative oncologist can balance that by offering a complementary treatment that could lower the risk.

Because savvy patients demand it, many of the best university cancer centers now have a blend of both conventional and integrative oncology. This partnership is best.

Prepare Your Hospital Nest for Healing

While there may be great variability in how you will feel and how quickly you will heal after surgery, the environment you are in as soon as you wake up can help you better recover. At least a week or two before your scheduled surgery, ask your family and friends to load up memorabilia, smile and laughter stimulators, and whatever you want to hear and see in your hospital room during healing. Imagine waking up and opening your eyes to photos of your wedding day, your best vacation, and so on. While great advances have been made to get patients home within a day or two of surgery, or even the same day, sometimes your stay will be longer. The longer you will be inside your hospital nest, the more you need to decorate it.

Dr. Bill's hospital healing memory. *I still remember waking up from my colon cancer surgery in 1997 in a room where my favorite music was playing and my favorite photos were taped to the wall as close to my bed as possible. I remember waking up to the sight of our family of fourteen all standing on a big sailboat we* *had rented for a family trip of a lifetime in the Caribbean, with the joyful knowl-edge that we had planned a similar sailing trip in two months. Replaying those memories rerouted my attention to the happy-memory center of my brain and away from the pain center.*

A Room with a View

Whether you're in the hospital healing from cancer surgery or complications from cancer, or healing at home but confined indoors, spend as much time as possible with your bed or chair facing a window, preferably one looking out on green space and nature scenes. A study from Japan proved what nurses have long observed: bigger windows promote better healing. The study compared two groups of surgical patients from the same hospital. Those whose beds faced a window with a garden or mountain view healed faster and left the hospital sooner than those whose beds faced a wall.

Thank-Yous Are Therapeutic

Cancer-care providers can be among the most stressed of all healthcare providers. The science is continually being upgraded, treatment needs to be very personalized, and the field is changing so fast that keeping on top of the latest research can be a struggle. While they enjoy the "helper's high" effect from their patients' good results, they also may suffer a bit of treatment anxiety, and second-guess themselves when the outcome isn't so favorable. For these reasons, thank-you notes, gifts, and other little nuggets that show your appreciation for their care will be greatly appreciated by them—and, as an added perk, will help you feel good too.

Helpful Healing Advice from Martha's Breast Cancer Surgeon, Dr. Anderson

The time after a cancer diagnosis can be many things: frightening, disorienting, disheartening, and even infuriating. However, it can also be a very valuable time, one that lays the foundation for surgery, treatment, and, hopefully, life after cancer.

While every patient's experience is different, cancer is never easy. However, you can optimize treatment outcomes, as pointed out in this book, by preparing your mind, body, and spirit.

Mind: Help It Become Your Biggest Asset

The research is clear: your mindset has a powerful influence on your cancer outcomes. For example, studies have shown that patients with significant preoperative anxiety and depression suffer from increased complications, increased length of stay, and increased readmission. Significant emotional stress has been shown to increase the risk for metastatic disease in breast cancer patients due to its immunosuppressive effects.

This doesn't mean one needs to "stay positive" all of the time, as that task is impossible. It is important to acknowledge the various feelings that come along with a cancer diagnosis and develop coping strategies to manage these feelings and avoid becoming overwhelmed with anxiety and depression.

Pre-surgery anxiety is often acute due to the nature of the diagnosis and disease and the act of undergoing surgery. It's not a normal event that we routinely encounter. The best thing you can do to help is develop a mindset for success and focus on preparation. Feeling swept along by the disease without knowing what lies ahead is a powerful source of anxiety. But you don't have to be a prisoner of your diagnosis or passive passenger in the process. You can, and should, be a partner in your treatment.

Educate yourself. Even though the information they find can sometimes be frightening, most people nevertheless find researching and knowing about their cancer, surgery, and what to expect during the treatment and recovery less stressful than not knowing. Your surgeon will also provide you with a lot of information about your disease and treatment course and should be willing to answer any questions that you have.

Plan ahead. Make sure that you get prepared ahead of time and consider making a checklist to help you organize what needs to be done. Some points to consider: setting up a recovery area with everything you may need close at hand, arranging transportation to and from the surgery, preparing meals ahead of time, arranging for people to assist you with day-to-day chores and activities, and building social support. There are a number of social media applications that can help you organize your social support for meals and transportation. Planning in advance not only gives you something to focus on besides your cancer, it eliminates the future anxiety leaving it to the days and hours before surgery can bring.

Trust your team. Hopefully you are confident in your surgeon; if not, there is nothing wrong with selecting another. You should feel like a team. Once you reach the day of the operation, I recommend letting go and trusting the process, from preop to postop and admission (if applicable). The people guiding it have been through this hundreds or thousands of times, and their goal is to help you be cancer free.

Use distraction. It's normal for some stress and anxiety to remain despite the preparation described above. Don't forget about continuing to do all the things that bring you joy, like reading, spending time with friends and family, volunteering, or whatever else works for you.

Body: Treat Your Body Well. It Is the Only One You Have.

Throughout this book, the importance of exercise and lifestyle for optimal health has been emphasized. Not surprisingly, exercise and lifestyle choices are also important for pre-surgery preparation, post-surgical recovery, and long-term outcomes.

Exercise. Think "pre-habilitation," or preparing your body for success. Starting appropriate strength training and aerobic exercise prior to surgery helps to prepare your heart, lungs, and muscles for optimal recovery.

Additional benefits of exercise include impacting cancer directly. One study noted that exercise prior to surgery positively altered breast cancer gene expression in a way that was associated with decreased inflammation and an upregulation of immunity, leading to an increase in natural killer cell infiltration in the cancer! Besides these pre-habilitation benefits, another study of more than 1300 patients showed that 150 minutes per week (i.e., just under 22 minutes per day) of moderate exercise before and after surgery reduced cancer recurrence by nearly 40 percent and reduced mortality by nearly 50 percent, assessed one year after surgery. After two years, recurrence was reduced by 55 percent and mortality by 68 percent. There are many other similar studies with similar results; the data supporting the importance of exercise in cancer outcomes is compelling.

If you do not regularly exercise, now is the time to start. While there are many types of exercise to choose from (for example, aerobic, resistance, strength, flexibility, balance, etc.), aerobic exercise has been shown to be most effective at reducing stress and anxiety. Fortunately, aerobic exercise is a broad category with a lot of variety, including brisk walking or jogging, swimming, cycling, organized aerobic programs like Zumba, and many more.

Once physical restrictions are lifted after surgery, getting active again is a significant, positive part of your recovery.

Lifestyle. Lifestyle factors that you control don't just affect your risk of getting cancer in the first place (approximately 42 percent of total cancer cases and 45 percent of cancer deaths in the United States are linked to lifestyle related risk factors, while 5–10 percent are a result of familial risk or inherited genetic mutation). They also affect recovery and long-term outcomes, regardless of whether your cancer resulted from lifestyle, environmental factors, or an inherited genetic mutation.

According to a study done at the Fred Hutchinson Cancer Research Center in 2009, two alcoholic drinks per day (postoperatively) doubles the risk of post-operative complications, and just one drink per day increases the risk of a second breast cancer by 90 percent. Obesity has been shown to increase the risk of a second breast cancer by 50 percent, and smoking by 120 percent. Smoking also significantly increases wound healing complication rates.

Consequently, reducing or eliminating smoking and alcohol can significantly optimize surgical success and long-term outcomes.

Nutrition. It is essential to provide your body with what it needs to optimize healing from surgery and decrease the risk of wound infection and associated complications. While a carefully designed healthy diet can provide all of the nutrients you need for this and more, it is also worth considering supplementation with nutraceuticals to ensure adequate amounts are consumed (though you should consult with your cancer specialist before taking any supplements, as they could interact poorly with prescribed medications). Basic considerations include the need for increased protein; vitamins A, B, C, and D; zinc; and omega-3 fatty acids to support healing. Increasing protein intake has been shown to have a positive influence on cell-mediated immunity and to combat the muscle loss associated with surgery and cancer treatment.

Spirit: Forgive Your Body. Getting Cancer Can Feel Like a Betrayal.

An underappreciated focus in working through diagnosis, treatment, and recovery is your spirit. Spirit usually refers to something bigger than our physical body—a vital force or higher power that drives us forward in life, usually in a positive and meaningful way. But spirit also encompasses qualities like hope, wisdom, courage, perseverance, and forgiveness. Maintaining and remembering your spirit can help keep you rooted in the windstorm of cancer diagnosis and treatment.

While no definitive studies have yet demonstrated improved outcomes based on spirit, maintaining hope has long been associated with better maintenance of cancer treatment regimens. That is, maintaining your mind and body is easier when you maintain your spirit.

But how can you do that?

It's different for everyone and usually involves a combination of things. Faith, family, friends, practicing gratitude, journaling, meditation, mindfulness, and sometimes support groups or professional counseling are all common cornerstones of spirit maintenance during cancer treatment and recovery. They can help lift us out of the trenches of our diagnosis and treatment to place our focus on the bigger picture. And focusing on the bigger picture can let our hope, wisdom, courage, perseverance, and even forgiveness reemerge.

Forgiveness is often an important component of recovery because getting cancer can feel like being betrayed by your body. Surgery can change the way your body looks or works, as with a mastectomy; you may need to mourn the loss of the way your body was and accept the way your body is now. Hopefully, one day, you can even celebrate it.

Few want to be faced with such a test of the spirit, but you can emerge on the other side of your treatment with hope, wisdom, courage, and more that will serve you in the future, whatever life throws your way!

Maria Anderson, MD, FACS
Surgical Breast Oncologist

Build Your Support Team

In addition to your *medical* team, another team you will need is supportive friends, loved ones, and cancer survivors and thrivers, especially those who had cancers similar to yours. Treasure your team!

Be selective. Try to select only those support team members who are positive and uplifting—who send you "good vibes."

Shield yourself from advice overload. It's usual for your loved ones to overwhelm you with recommendations such as "try this supplement," and so on. First, process the treatment plan your oncologist gives you. Then, gradually let in other suggestions from your support team—in particular from those who can share with you tools they learned while healing their own cancer.

The Benefits of Having a Cancer-Healing Mindset and Wisely Partnering with Your Oncologist

Science says that people with cancer who enjoy this mindset and partnership are more likely to experience:

- More confidence and calm during treatment
- Less anxiety and depression
- Reduced fear of cancer recurrence
- Better ability to manage emotions
- Better decision-making
- A healthier, smarter immune system
- Less pain, and better results from pharmacological pain relievers
- Better healing after surgery
- Faster wound healing

- Better healing of tissues affected by cancer or cancer treatment
- Better support from family and friends
- Fewer intestinal upsets
- Less fatigue
- Reduced cancer-treatment bills
- Improved partnership with caregivers
- Increased survival rate
- Better quality of life

Our Cancer-Healing Wish

Imagine you are consulting with your chosen oncologist, who, after outlining your personalized treatment plan, says, "Besides what I can do for you, here's what *you* can do to help yourself heal," and hands you a copy of this book.

Cancer is an "inside problem." Transformation is an "inside solution." In cancer healing we prefer the deeper term "transformation" to "change." Since cancer is an imbalance deep inside your body's cells, you need a transformation from deep within your body—not just new "habits" but new *cravings* that automatically prompt you to be the new, healthier you.

Wisely partnering with your cancer-care providers isn't just about your medical treatment. It's about supporting their work with what you do at home, too, with the self-help skills you will now learn in Part III.

Part III

How to L.E.A.N. into Cancer Healing

L.E.A.N. (*l*ifestyle, *e*xercise, *a*ttitude, and *n*utrition) is the motivational term we have used in our medical practice for over twenty years. How you live, move, think, and eat greatly affects how well you heal, which is true for cancer as much as any other disease. The tools to help heal yourself from cancer that you will read—and use—in this next part of the book are supported by science and based on our twenty-five years of personal and medical experience.

Chapter 5

Eat Our Eight-Part Conquer-Cancer Diet

Want to feel healthier, sooner? Dive right into our cancer-conquering way of eating.

The foods we highlight here, and how we recommend eating them, help speed healing and prevent future cancer by:

- Preventing the malnutrition that often accompanies cancer treatments and healing.
- Helping your immune system fight smarter.
- Reducing foods that feed cancer.
- Creating super-synergy with the rest of our conquer-cancer program.

By following the eight parts of our conquer-cancer diet, you will *transform your tastes* from experiencing "don't like, but must eat" to liking this new cancer-conquering way of eating, to *craving* it. After a few weeks of conquer-cancer eating, the *wisdom of the body,* your inner prompts, clicks in to tell you, "Finally, you're eating the way your body was designed. Keep it up!"

"Good gut feelings" are often the first feel-good effect. You may feel more energy and more mental clarity. Your immune system will get smarter. Imagine your immune-system army prompting you: "You're feeding us better so we'll fight better for you." And, if your chemotherapy pills could talk, they would shout, "Eat better, and we'll work better for you!" (For a detailed explanation of what's going on inside during your "transformation," see *The Dr. Sears T5 Wellness Plan*.)

> ## The smarter your meal, the better you heal.

The key to conquer-cancer eating is simple:

1. Do eat foods that fight cancer cells.
2. Don't eat foods that feed cancer cells.

Consider this chapter your crash course in *nutritional oncology*. Eat cancer away before it eats you away!

How food fights or feeds cancer. Because they multiply so fast, cancer cells are ravenous eaters. Cancer can only spread if its cells have what they need to grow.

Imagine a conference of cancer cells getting together to design the diet they like. After hearing from each cell what their favorite foods are, the biggest and baddest cancer cell concludes: "We don't have to design a new diet to feed us, we've already got one—the standard American diet (SAD)."

Cancer cells crave carbs. They love high blood sugar spikes. The SAD is high in carbs that spike blood sugar.

Let's compare the SAD to the conquer-cancer diet (CCD) you'll learn in this chapter:

How SAD Feeds Cancer	How Our CCD Fights (and Prevents) Cancer
• High in added sugar	• Low in added sugar
• Low in antioxidants	• High in antioxidants
• High in animal-based foods, low in plant-based foods	• High in plant-based foods, low in animal-based foods
• Low in fiber	• High in fiber
• High in chemical food additives that throw the immune system out of balance	• Rich in real foods that promote immune system balance
• Has an omega imbalance: high in omega-6 fats, low in omega-3 fats	• Has a smart balance of omega-3 and omega-6 fats
• Encourages gorging, which results in sugar spikes	• Encourages grazing, which balances blood sugar
• Less filling, so you eat more	• More filling, so you naturally eat less
• Tainted with carcinogenic pesticides	• Cleaner—fewer carcinogens

Grow your conquer-cancer garden inside. Cancer cells grow and spread when the soil they're in is fertile, or cancer-friendly. The SAD diet is like adding chemical fertilizers to a cancer garden. Eating a cancer-healing diet starts with leaving out what cancer craves, by eating smarter and lower carb.

When Bill had his first cancer back in 1997, the conventional wisdom was *low-fat* and *high-carb* eating. Science has since revealed that fad was a *big, fat, sweet lie*. You don't get fat by eating smart fats. You get fat by eating dumb carbs. And when you take the fat out of food, you have to fill your diet with more carbs to get enough calories.

Replacing healthy fats (see page 210) with unhealthy carbs gives you a double fault that fuels more cancer. Supporting the ISA lesson "Feed us well and we'll fight better for you," smart fats smarten the cancer-fighting NK cell's cell membrane, which is mostly made of fat, by making it more selective and protective. Remember our mantra: "Every organ of the body is only as healthy as its cells, and every cell is only as healthy as the membrane protecting it." Could a low-fat, high cancer-feeding diet weaken cell membranes, and therefore NK cells? We believe so.

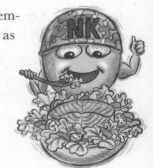

You can remember a cancer-feeding carb by the four Fs: it's *fake*, *fast*, *fiberless*, and *factory-made*.

Chemo Prevention

This delicious buzzword among integrative oncologists refers to how certain nutrients you eat (as well as the lifestyle choices you make) help prevent cancer, lessen adverse effects of conventional cancer treatment, and improve cancer healing. Think of our conquer-cancer diet as preventative chemotherapy. Does that sound like a "medicine" you want to take?

Get ready to eat your way to less cancer!

1. Think Before You Eat

Smart conquer-cancer eating begins in your brain. Changing your thoughts gradually grows your food-craving areas for conquer-cancer foods and shrinks your craving areas for feed-cancer foods.

Here's how to transform your tastes by think-changing your cravings. Before you reach for that sugar-infected doughnut, dwell on the thought: "Will this food feed or starve my cancer?" Visualize a cancer cell in your body saying, "Yum, like!"

Practice makes conquer-cancer thoughts perfect. Your rational brain and your pleasure centers will constantly battle each other. You may rationalize, "Oh, that doughnut will make me so happy! And decreasing stress can decrease my cancer risk." Instead train yourself to think, "Don't go there, brain; I'm smarter than that!"

Dr. Bill shares: *Here's what helped me stick to a lifesaving and cancer-fighting way of eating: when I would have a weak moment and crave carbs, to get me onto a healthier craving path I would imagine a cancer cell in my body smiling and saying, "Yum! Feed me those fake and fast carbs and I'll grow and multiply fast."*

I also had to do a bit of preprogramming my brain to "like" the foods that were best for me. One of my least favorite foods was broccoli. As I ate it, I would imagine the broccoli feeding my conquer-cancer army inside, as I repeated the refrain, "I know they're so good for me . . ." Over a period of a few weeks to a few months I gradually noticed a change from "don't like, but must eat" to "like a little" to "like a lot," to finally "crave."

2. Eat More Conquer-Cancer Foods

To grow the crave-real-food center in your brain, let's now learn about science-supported conquer-cancer foods.

The double whammy of conquer-cancer foods. Many of the foods in this section not only have direct anti-cancer cell effects, but also are the favorite foods of your cancer-fighting army inside, helping you to achieve the double goal:

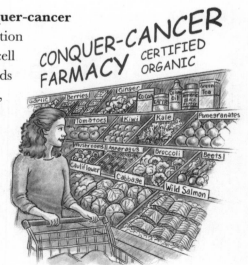

- Help keep normal cells from becoming cancerous.
- Kill those renegades that do become cancer cells.

This helps prevent the cancer you have from spreading and new cancer from developing.

Science-Supported Conquer-Cancer Foods

Foods that science says help fight cancer enjoy all or most of the following four features:

- Low in added sugar
- High in fiber, slow-release carbs, antioxidants, and other cancer-fighting biochemicals
- High in smart nutrients for your brain and ISA
- Promote leanness instead of obesity

We have chosen the following foods because they have these conquer-cancer biochemical effects:

- Artichokes
- Asparagus
- Beets
- Beet greens
- Berries, especially blueberries, tart cherries, strawberries, raspberries, cranberries
- Broccoli
- Brussels sprouts
- Cabbage
- Capers
- Cauliflower
- Chili peppers
- Cocoa
- Garlic
- Ginger
- Kale
- Kiwi
- Leeks
- Lemons
- Mushrooms, especially shiitake, chaga, reishi
- Olive oil
- Onions
- Pomegranates
- Radishes
- Salmon (wild, not farmed)
- Scallions
- Spinach
- Tomatoes
- Turmeric and black pepper

More color, less cancer. Remember Mom's advice to "Put more color on your plate"? Dr. Mom was right. Our conquer-cancer plate is color-*full*. The nutrients, called antioxidants, that give foods their color are also the ones that fight cancer best. And the deeper the color, usually the richer the antioxidant content of the food.

> Think: *awesome antioxidants against awful cancer.*

When you hear the term "antioxidants," think "anti-cancer." Here's why.

As your cells do their job as the energy-producing batteries of your body, they produce "exhaust," aka *oxidants*, that can damage cell metabolism and upset the cell's balance (cancer is a cell out of biochemical balance). Excess oxidants also cause wear and tear on the cell that affects cell health and is one of the basic causes of aging. Oxidants age you! Excess oxidants can also trigger DNA mutation, a root cause of cancer.

Enter *antioxidants*. Antioxidants help protect DNA from these excess oxidant attacks. These beautiful biochemicals in colorful foods—blue, red, green, yellow, orange, and purple—both slow your aging and help you prevent and heal from cancer.

A Second Helping of Conquer-Cancer Foods

Many of the following foods, while not as directly cancer-conquering as the list on page 84, also help build a healthier brain and immune system, your two partners in cancer healing:

- Animal-based foods, such as meat and eggs (when organic, free-range, and 100 percent grass-fed and grass-finished). Keep these to no more than 10 to 20 percent of your average daily diet.
- Dark chocolate (80 to 85 percent cacao).

- Flax oil (not a substitute for fish oil).
- Kefir and yogurt (when organic, grass-fed, unsweetened, and whole milk).
- Medium-chain triglycerides (MCT) oil or coconut oil (a tablespoon a day).
- Lemon and lime peels (organic). These are great in smoothies.
- Raw nuts and seeds, especially raw almonds, raw Brazil nuts, and raw pumpkin seeds.

If possible, eat all organic fruits and vegetables to avoid carcinogenic pesticides (see ewg.org for lists of the "Dirty Dozen" and the "Clean Fifteen").

Eat real! Love how you feel!

The Top Conquer-Cancer Food

Become a sea-foodie. Our top CCF pick is . . . (drums rolling) . . . wild salmon, for two reasons: It makes sense, and it's supported by science.

Cancer and chemotherapy are frequently accompanied by malnutrition. Wild salmon is the most nutrient-dense food you can eat. It also contains more conquer-cancer nutrients—namely omega-3 DHA and EPA, vitamin D, astaxanthin, selenium, choline, vitamin B6, vitamin B12, and tryptophan—per calorie than any other food.

Omega-3 fats, the top nutrient in wild salmon, is the nutrient supported by the most science. Here's a summary of what seafood science says:

- The European Prospective Investigation into Cancer (EPIC), one of the largest "eat more fish, get less cancer" studies, analyzed the dietary habits of thousands of people from ten

European countries. Those who ate 10 to 20 ounces of seafood per week were significantly less likely to get colon cancer.

- Another study showed that people who ate the most *fatty fish* got less cancer, especially oral cancers, melanoma, pancreatic, colon, prostate, uterine, and breast cancers.

Seafood's conquer-cancer effect seems to happen at the cellular level. As you learned on page 26, a healthy cell becomes a renegade cancer cell when it grows and multiplies out of control. Omega-3s help regulate the genes inside cells that control cell growth. Imagine an omega-3 molecule saying to a cellular growth gene, "Grow smart, grow safely. Then, when you've finished your job, retire and make room for a younger and healthier cell" (see apoptosis, page 26). Or, imagine a molecule, let's call her Dr. O. Mega III, as an intracellular cancer doctor, prescribing DHA and EPA and saying, "Eat this, get less cancer." Omega-3s also "down-regulate," or balance, the blood level of pro-inflammatory (pro-cancer) biochemicals such as COX-2 and prostaglandins that result from the SAD way of eating and can act as fertilizers for cancer cells.

If you are not yet motivated to think, "I want more omega-3s inside my cells and bloodstream," read on. The healthier a cell is, the less chance it has of becoming cancerous. The healthier the cell membrane, the healthier the entire cell. Omega-3s are the most important nutrient for healthier cell membranes. They are the smart fats you learned about on page 81 that help cell membranes become more selective and protective. That's just what you want for cellular health: membranes that let cancer-fighters in, and keep cancer-causers out.

Dr. Bill shares: *While I wasn't initially fond of fish, to heal from my first cancer I became a sea-foodie by mastering the conquer-cancer mindset of "I must eat this food and learn to like it. Do I need it to heal from cancer and prevent more cancer? Yes! Therefore, I will eat it." It's amazing how your mind can take charge of your food choices when you teach it to.* (See more, pages 82–83.)

Omega imbalance contributes to cancer. On page 81, you learned why immune system imbalance and obesity are top cancer contributors.

When the omega-6/omega-3 ratio in our diet averages around 2:1, our immune system is in better balance and our body tends to be leaner. Yet, the *oiling of the American diet* has added cheaper omega-6 fats (such as corn and cottonseed oils) to our daily eating, contributing to ratios as high as 10:1 or even 20:1, as Americans have gotten fatter, suffered more "-itis" illnesses, and gotten more cancer.

Conquer-Cancer Effects of Seafood-Based Omega-3s

Here's a summary of what these magnificent molecules can do for you:

- Protect cell membranes.
- Keep genes from going haywire and becoming cancer-promoting.
- Reduce cancer-causing inflammatory biochemicals.
- Smarten the immune system to better fight cancer.
- Regulate cell growth.

Because it's full of what's called the "merry omegas," seafood is also mood food. Depression frequently accompanies cancer. Studies show that omega-3s lift up your mood.

(For more information about omega-3s, see our conquer cancer reading list, pages 216–221.)

"Currently, the biggest nutritional deficiency in Western industrialized countries is the low intake of omega-3 fatty acids."
—Richard Béliveau and Denis Gingras,
Foods That Fight Cancer: Preventing Cancer Through Diet

Don't be *fish-fooled!* When possible, *go wild!* When purchasing fish, pay attention to the label. "Organic" could mean the fish were still *farmed*, yet fed "organic" grains, which can result in a higher and more pro-inflammatory omega-6/omega-3 ratio than is present in wild seafood.

Tips for eating sufficient conquer-cancer seafood:

- Eat at least two fist-size portions (around 12 ounces) of wild Pacific salmon a week.
- Caviar and salmon roe (fish eggs) are the richest source of omega-3 DHA and EPA per ounce.

Salmon says, "Read more about me!" Enjoy a free download of Dr. Bill's forty-two–page storybook *Salmon Says*: vitalchoice.com/content/salmonsays.

Measure Your Omegas

How do you know if you have enough cancer-fighting omega-3s in your bloodstream? Measure your omega-3 blood levels. It's not how much of a nutrient you eat that counts, but rather how much of that nutrient your intestines *absorb*, and that amount can be as individual as your cancer cells. You may be a low absorber or a high absorber. Using a simple fingerstick test that uses one drop of blood to measure the percentage of omega fats in your red blood cell membranes gives you a clue of whether you have an "omega-3 sufficiency" or an "omega-3 insufficiency." Strive for an omega-3 index above 8 percent. See AskDrSears.com/omega-3index for where to get a test and how to use it.

3. Eat Fewer Dumb Carbs

Besides eating more healthy fats, eating fewer dumb carbs may be the smartest conquer-cancer eating change you can make. Here's how I explain smart sugars and dumb sugars to kids with cancer:

"A smart sugar plays with its friends: protein, fat, and fiber. It never plays alone. Picture the sugar holding hands with its friends as it travels down through your gut. The friends grab on to the sugar and keep it from being absorbed too fast, so you don't get sugar spikes." ("Avoid sugar spikes" is Conquer-Cancer Eating 101.) "A dumb sugar, on the other hand, such as a sugar-sweetened soda, has no friends. When you guzzle it, your blood sugar spikes and your cancer cells yell: 'Here comes my favorite food!'"

Cancer specialists estimate that 80 percent of cancers are caused or worsened by these sugar spikes, because sugar spikes trigger a top cancer cell fertilizer called insulin growth factor (IGF). Scientists also believe that these *spikes* may be more cancer-causing than the actual number of grams of sugar you eat—which is why the company the sugar keeps (fat, fiber, and protein) is so important.

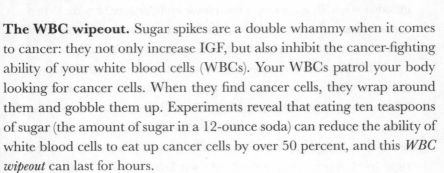

The WBC wipeout. Sugar spikes are a double whammy when it comes to cancer: they not only increase IGF, but also inhibit the cancer-fighting ability of your white blood cells (WBCs). Your WBCs patrol your body looking for cancer cells. When they find cancer cells, they wrap around them and gobble them up. Experiments reveal that eating ten teaspoons of sugar (the amount of sugar in a 12-ounce soda) can reduce the ability of white blood cells to eat up cancer cells by over 50 percent, and this *WBC wipeout* can last for hours.

Sugar Shows Where Your Cancer Is

Suppose you scheduled an X-ray at your friendly neighborhood radiology lab. You ask the doctor, "What do you have to inject into my body to find out where my cancer is and how fast it might be growing?" The doctor answers: "Sugar!" In a PET scan designed to detect cancer, radioactive glucose is injected into a patient's veins. Since cancer cells gobble up the glucose much faster than healthy cells do, they light up faster on the screen.

Here's a second helping at the cellular level of how sugar feeds cancer: High sugar spikes create more *insulin receptors* on the surfaces of healthy cells, which is sort of like adding more doors to allow glucose to enter faster. This enables potential cancer cells to consume blood sugar fifty times faster than normal cells. Remember, cancer cells crave sugar.

Your Conquer-Cancer Symphony Inside

In several of our recent books we talk about how health is like your body's symphony orchestra: it requires all of your endocrine glands to play in harmony, or what we call *hormonal health.* When there is hormonal disharmony, unmelodious music—in this case, cancer—can result. *Cancer is a disease of hormonal disharmony.*

Which hormone makes the most difference in whether your hormonal symphony orchestra plays the harmonious music of health or unharmonious music of cancer? The answer is one of the body's master conductors—insulin. Like a conductor, who must remain on tempo at all times, insulin that is consistently at the right level deprives cancer cells of their favorite food, sugar. This has led to one of the simplest preventive medicines for cancer, heart disease, and many other diseases: *stable blood insulin levels.*

It just so happens that the increase in cancer rates have paralleled the increase in type 2 diabetes (excess insulin levels). Any correlation? We think so.

Not so sweet. Many doctors wisely believe that the rise in added sugar in the SAD (standard American diet) over the past fifty years correlates with an increase in cancer. This conviction led to one of the best label-law changes in history, requiring nutrition labels to include "grams of added sugar." You'll now often see "no added sugar" touted on the front of food labels. This push for less added sugar in foods can be a mixed blessing, however. Yes, no added sugar is good for cancer healing and prevention, yet replacing added sugars with artificial sweeteners is not.

Your New Conquer-Cancer Food Math

Our mantra, "Avoid sugar spikes," is the basis of our conquer-cancer diet:

- Eat a lot more healthy fats.
- Eat a little more healthy protein.
- Eat a lot fewer dumb carbs.

Healthy fats don't spike blood insulin levels. Proteins may, but only a little. Carbs spike a lot.

In short, smart fats are cancer's foe. Dumb carbs are cancer's friend. How do you want your cancer cells to feel about your diet—"yuck" or "yum"? The choice is yours.

Fast carbs versus slow carbs. The more slowly your intestines absorb a carbohydrate, the less it becomes a favorite cancer-feeding food. Ever wonder why your intestines are so long, around twenty-five feet? One reason, we believe, is because your intestines like "slow carbs"—real foods in which carbs are partnered with fat, protein, and fiber. Your intestines are longer so they can take longer to digest and absorb carbs, so those carbs *spike less*. Your conquer-cancer army inside likes that! "Fast carbs" go fast into your bloodstream—spike! Cancer cells like that. Again, fast carbs feed cancer; slow carbs don't.

Vegetables are smart carbs. Our conquer-cancer diet is a "right-carb" and "slow-carb" diet more than a "low-carb" one. That's why most vegetables are "free foods" in all anti-cancer diets. Their bulk is mostly water and fiber. They're *chewy* so you eat them more slowly, digest them more slowly, and absorb their natural sugars more slowly. No sugar spikes!

Dr. Bill advises: *Eat fewer carbs at your last meal. You are more likely to burn rather than store the carbs you eat earlier in the day.*

What's the worst food you can eat that cancer cells like? Imagine a group of "fats scientists," "sugar scientists," and cancer specialists getting together to vote on the worst cancer-promoting food or drink. Which of these would be the winner (or really the loser):

a. A hamburger
b. Mom's apple pie
c. A cola

Answer: The cola. Sugar water feeds cancer (though note that artificial sweeteners may be even worse). The sugar spikes it causes feed excess belly fat, a storage bank for cancer-feeding chemicals. And colas teach your crave center to tell you to drink more—meaning cancer cells grow more. Your heart, brain, and conquer-cancer army inside vote to chuck sodas.

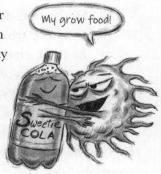

A Tale of Two Carbies

Chuck guzzles a cola. Because sweetened beverages are basically sugar water (plus artificial coloring, another cancer contributor), the sugar rushes into Chuck's blood, causing a sugar spike. His cancer cells say, "Yum, a feast! We're going to grow and multiply."

Suzy eats a salad. Because the carbs in a chewy vegetable salad are naturally partnered with fiber, protein, and fats, the carbs are absorbed very slowly into her bloodstream. No spikes, no cancer feeding. And when cancer cells go hungry, they either die or go to sleep and stop multiplying.

Bitter is better. Cancer-prevention specialists have long taught that the more bitter a food, the more anti-cancer power it has. An example is how arugula is a more powerful cancer-calmer than regular lettuce.

Generally, bitter taste correlates with high antioxidant (cancer-fighting) content, as in the following anti-cancer foods: dark chocolate (85 percent cocoa), bitter herbs like thyme and rosemary, lemon peel, arugula, and garlic.

Transform Your Tastes

After eating our conquer-cancer diet for a month or two, your tastes will transform toward healing, as you imprint "This is how I must eat" and "This is how I will eat" in your conquer-cancer mind until finally your brain thinks, "These are the foods I *crave* to eat."

Can conquer-cancer eating change your mind? After a few months of eating our conquer-cancer diet, Dr. Bill noticed a mindset change. While shopping in a supermarket or looking at a restaurant buffet, he noticed his eyes were magnetically drawn to focus more on the conquer-cancer foods, mainly those that were the most colorful. He believes he had planted a color-craving conquer-cancer food section in his mind. He smiled and felt pleasant feelings when looking at the healthier foods, and when he looked at junk foods, he cringed. His mind was already intuitively separating "like" from "don't like."

Science agrees. A fascinating study from Tufts University had volunteers eat mainly the foods in our conquer-cancer diet, those naturally low in sugar and higher in protein, fiber, and healthy fats. Brain scans in these healthy eaters showed their pleasure centers automatically lit up more when they viewed pictures of the healthy foods they were eating than when they viewed pictures of junk foods.

A tip from chocolate-loving cancer survivor Dr. Bill. *When I was transforming my diet, the hardest no-no for me to give up was chocolate. I knew that the higher the percentage of cocoa in a piece of chocolate, the higher its antioxidant content, and antioxidants are anti-cancer. Yet, bittersweetly, the higher the percentage of cocoa, the lower the added sugar, and the more bitter the taste.*

Here's how my transformation worked, and you can do the same. Eat a square of dark chocolate with 60 percent cocoa daily for a week. Then, each week for the next five weeks, increase the cocoa content by 5 percent until you get to the healthful 80 to 85 percent cocoa. At first, I had to constantly remind myself that "bitter was better" for fighting cancer, but by the end of the five weeks, I enjoyed the dark chocolate with 85 percent cocoa, and the square of the 60 percent tasted way too sweet and even unpleasant. The smart center in my brain won!

Not everyone can buy into "the bitter, the better" concept, especially right away. If you are still craving something sweet, there are some good and bad compromises.

Artificial sweeteners and chemical flavor-enhancers are on the "naughty list." Coconut palm sugar, cinnamon, raw organic cocoa, and diced fruits are on the "nice list." Dr. Bill occasionally sweetens his coffee with a smashed banana. It took a while to get used to, but now he enjoys it as much as a spoonful of sugar. And to give a tangy taste to his morning smoothie, he sometimes adds a pinch of stevia. "Sweet" is not synonymous with added sugar.

Of course, a spoonful of sugar won't "cause" cancer, yet all those daily "contributors" such as SAD, sitting more than moving, being stressed out, toxin exposure, and so on can add up to cancer. So, it makes sense to omit, or lessen, as many of these contributors as you can—beginning with a top contributor, added table sugar.

Less Alcohol, Less Cancer

If you enjoy an occasional drink, do you need to stop to heal from cancer? Not necessarily!

On first glance, it makes sense to give up all alcohol while healing from your cancer. Sugar spikes are a top cancer feeder, and alcohol is a top sugar spiker. In fact, alcohol has a unique carb-spiking quirk. Unlike other sugars, it can eat its way through the protective mucus lining of your stomach to quickly get into your bloodstream. There, it spikes blood sugar more than other sugars, which are absorbed more slowly through your intestines.

In addition, alcohol can contribute to cancer in these ways:

- It weakens the immune system.
- It throws inflammation out of balance. Inflammation imbalance feeds cancer.
- It weakens the liver—your primary detox organ for carcinogens.
- It can contribute to deficiencies of nutrients such as folate.
- It sabotages cancer-healing sleep (see why quality sleep is good "medicine" for cancer-healing in Chapter 8).

It's not always that easy to give up alcohol, however. Nor do we believe it is absolutely necessary. Instead of "Don't drink!" we advise, "If you choose to drink, drink smart!"

Our recipe for smart drinking:

- Never drink alcohol on an empty stomach. Instead, sip slowly with meals, and delay your first sip until you're at least a quarter into your meal to let the food slow the absorption of the alcohol.
- Pair your alcohol with a raw, multi-vegetable salad to lessen possible nutrient deficiencies.
- Choose red wine over hard liquors, which are much higher in fast-absorbing carbs. Be sure it's certified organic to avoid pesticides.
- Drink no more than one glass a meal, and no more than three times a week.

For an in-depth discussion on how to drink smart, see *The Healthy Brain Book.*

4. Grazing Is Great for Cancer Prevention and Healing

As we've shown, "avoid sugar spikes" is Conquer-Cancer Eating 101. Gorgers spike; grazers don't. It's as simple and as healthy as that!

The smaller your meal, the better you heal.

Switching to grazing makes sense for two reasons:

1. Grazers don't get sugar and insulin spikes. They enjoy lower blood levels of these two cancer fertilizers.

2. Grazers are usually leaner than gorgers. Obesity is the top contributor to cancer.

Grazers also enjoy a lower incidence of not just cancer, but also just about every disease you don't want to get, from type 2 diabetes to cardiovascular disease.

Graze to the "rule of twos." This is one of the most popular teachings in our Dr. Sears Wellness Institute coaching classes. Healthy cells like a steady supply of carbohydrates; cancer cells like sugar spikes. Keeping in mind how eating too much too fast leads to sugar and insulin spikes that fuel cancer growth, to spike less and get cancer less, follow these rules:

- Eat *twice* as often.
- Eat *half* as much.
- Chew *twice* as long.
- Take *twice* the time to dine.

The "rule of twos" is especially helpful to prevent one of the top malignancies: colon cancer. That makes sense because the more work the upper part of your intestines does during eating and digesting, the less the lower part of your digestive tract is overworked. Think of chewing as your food blender. Colons like that. The better digestive efforts you make at the top of your GI tract, the less wear and tear—and cancer—on the bottom end.

Are You a Sugar Spiker? How to Tell

Measure your blood sugar! Since no one conquer-cancer diet fits all, and your top goal is to blunt blood sugar spikes, *get a glucometer.* In consultation with your doctor, wear it, read it, and personalize your conquer-cancer diet as needed to keep your blood sugar levels reasonably steady throughout the day. It can help to journal what you're eating and what you're seeing on the glucometer in response.

> **Dr. Bill's sugar story.** *After a few months of transforming from a gorger to a grazer, I started measuring my blood sugar every couple hours while awake and noticed I had transformed from being "spiky" to being "steady."*

Chew cancer away. Besides balancing your blood sugar, chewing on certain crunchy vegetables, such as broccoli, releases more of a powerful phytonutrient they contain, called sulforaphane. Remember, *phytos fight cancer.* As you're chewing on a broccoli floret, imagine: "I'm opening a box of anti-cancer medicines in the broccoli so they can benefit my body." You also must "press" (chew) garlic to release its anti-cancer medicine, called allicin.

Both children and medical doctors enjoy potty talk, so another way I get people of all ages to remember to "chew-chew times two" is to think, "The better you chew, the better you poo!" Stools that are too large, too hard, and too infrequent can set up your colon lining for cancer. My patients would report that once they went from being a gorger to being a grazer, and ate according to the rule of twos, the number of their bowel movements at least doubled in frequency and softened in consistency—just what colon-cancer prevention needs.

Water your cancer away. You want to make sure you're drinking *at least* ½ ounce of water per pound of body weight each day. Yet, in addition to drinking your water, *eat more water.* Water-rich plant foods, especially veggies, have higher fiber and are eaten more slowly, which helps you feel fuller faster, in addition to helping soften your stools.

Cooking Cancer Away

It's not only the foods you eat but how you cook them that can contribute to cancer. Dr. Bill's many years of steak and burger ordering—"Burn a big one for me, Bud!"—probably contributed to his colon cancer. Grilling over high heat, such as charbroiling or flame-cooking meat until it is well done, can release carcinogens into the meat called heterocyclic amines (HCAs), which over time can accumulate in tissues, damage cellular DNA, and trigger cancer. Years of eating overcooked meats can eventually overwhelm your natural cellular detox system, causing it to cry, "Enough already! We're damaged and becoming cancer cells."

Follow these conquer-cancer cooking tips:

- Cook low and slow. This not only reduces HCAs but also preserves more nutrients.
- To reduce the chemical contributors to cancer from overcooked meat, enjoy poaching, stewing, slow-cooking at low heat, steam-cooking, or pressure-cooking instead. We still enjoy our meat (wild game, grass-fed meats, and organic chicken), but we *wet-sauté* it (we use half avocado oil and half hot water to steam and sauté the meat until done) or slow-cook it in a Crockpot.
- Marinate your meat. Marinating can lessen HCA production. (We make our own marinade with lemon juice, Dijon mustard, garlic, rosemary, and avocado oil.)
- When cooking fish, begin with the skin side down. This self-marinates the fatty side and lessens the cooking time of the other side.
- Pair meat with vegetables. Suppose you are invited to a barbecue and off the flame comes a blackened piece of beef—to be polite you nibble a bit. Adding several large servings of two big anti-cancer "Bs," broccoli and

Brussels sprouts, mutes some of the HCAs from the charred meat.

In the book he coauthored with Donald Abrams, *Integrative Oncology,* Dr. Andrew Weil summarized it well: "The higher the temperature and the longer the cooking time, the higher the dose of carcinogens."

Remember: Cooking can be carcinogenic. You can change that!

5. Burn More Than You Eat

One of Dr. Bill's favorite age-well tools is to burn more calories than he eats—at least 20 percent more. On average, he eats around 2,200 calories a day, but burns around 2,500 to 2,700 calories. Some cancer specialists recommend even more caloric restriction (CR), as well as something you may have heard of called intermittent fasting (IF) (see page 103).

The theory behind the "fewer calories, less cancer" is that during fasting, the level of cancer-feeding biochemicals in your blood, such as IGF-1, glucose, and insulin, go down. Burning more calories than you eat also lessens cellular and tissue inflammation and oxidation, which contribute to cancer (see page 116).

Science agrees. Even though most of these studies on caloric restriction were done on animals, usually rats and mice, there are also enough human studies supporting that it works. It also just makes sense. A person eating less than they burn is more likely to decrease the top contributors to cancer: obesity, excess belly fat, blood sugar spikes, and inflammation. And as an added health perk, our "burn more than you eat" advice has been shown to prompt your NK cells to fight better for you.

Calorie *counting* is less important for anti-cancer eating. How a food affects your hormonal harmony—whether it makes your blood glucose steady or spiky—is much more important than how many calories it contains. Focus on eating *nutrient-dense* foods (foods with more conquer-cancer nutrients per calorie) regardless of calories, and avoid foods with fewer nutrients per calorie.

To start eating less, burning more, and conquer your cancer:

1. Eat a diet rich in the conquer-cancer foods listed on page 84. Gradually you will feel fuller faster and naturally eat less—a perk of eating more slowly and chewing longer, too.
2. Gradually increase your daily amount of exercise until you are burning more calories than you eat.

If you are already obese with extra belly fat, then yes, you must work out your personal "burn more than you eat" plan. But otherwise, if you are exercising more and also notice you are naturally eating less, you probably don't need to count calories.

Martha notes: *Please don't get anxious about counting calories and getting all our conquer-cancer food rules right! Anxiety feeds cancer, too. Beginning "burn more than you eat" cancer healers may need to count calories for a while, but eventually, as your body resets its* appe-stat *(like a thermostat for your appetite), you will naturally eat fewer calories than you burn.*

During my cancer healing I gave in to my comfort-food treats without anxiety or regrets. Eventually, I tamed those treats to never more than 10 percent of my daily calories and gradually even reduced my cravings for them.

Your body, the most adaptable and resilient machine ever made, will automatically reprogram its metabolism to make it more fuel efficient. Just as a fuel-efficient car that runs on cleaner-burning fuel lasts longer, your body will also last longer. You'll get "more miles per gallon" (more energy from less fuel-burning) and see less wear and tear (less oxidation and inflammation, which lowers the carcinogenic effects on cells). These fuel changes also make the cells of your body healthier and more resistant to disease. And remember what you learned earlier: every tissue of your body is only as healthy as the cells it comprises.

Intermittent Fasting and Ketogenic Diets

I've heard that intermittent fasting and ketogenic diets can help treat cancer. How does this work?

"Fasting" simply means going without food and drinking only water for a length of time, anywhere from the usual twelve-hour fast between dinner and breakfast to something longer, say fourteen or sixteen hours, to a full day. "Intermittent" means you make two choices—how many hours to fast and which days to fast—and on the remaining days resume your normal, and hopefully healthy, eating habits. Oftentimes, intermittent fasting is paired with *caloric restriction* (CR). For example, you may choose two days each week to eat much less, say only 600 to 700 calories per day. Those would be your intermittent fasting days. On the other five days, you would eat as you normally do.

Intermittent fasting (IF) has long been known to help treat and prevent type 2 diabetes, metabolic syndrome, and other illnesses related to excess belly fat, and it makes sense that any change in eating habits that reduces obesity, especially excess belly fat, can help you prevent and heal from cancer. Remember, fasting starves cancer cells but not healthy cells. (See "The Leaner You Are, the Less Cancer You Are Likely to Get" on page 121.)

But there is also a cellular mechanism that helps explain why intermittent fasting can help treat cancer. By eating less, you dial down the metabolic rate of cells, which in turn lessens their likelihood of turning cancerous. Simply put, when you intermittently fast, the body runs out of its usual fuel, glucose (most of us have a twelve-hour supply in our glucose fuel tank, our liver), which cancer cells love, and starts breaking down its reserve fuel (fats) into *ketones*, an alternative fuel source for the body and brain that starves cancer cells. This is also the basis for using a ketogenic diet to fight cancer: when you eat fewer carbs, your body, especially your brain, automatically switches its fuel from sugar to ketones—a cleaner and more efficient energy source that also starves cancer cells.

Before deciding to do IF, CR, keto, or any other way of eating, be sure to personalize it with consultation from nutrition-savvy healthcare providers.

6. Enjoy the Sipping Solution

"Gut upsets" top the side effects list for both cancer-related anxiety and cancer treatment, especially chemo. So, early on, focus on eating foods that give you good gut feelings. Usually this begins with three simple changes:

1. Eat the most gut-friendly foods, which your *"eat this–feel this"* gut feedback will tell you.
2. Eat according to the "rule of twos." You just learned why and how on page 98.
3. Enjoy the sipping solution.

Dr. Bill's story. *During my healing from the gut-unfriendly trio of surgery, chemo, and radiation therapy for my colon cancer, I reasoned:*

-   *If I can make the work of digestion easier by what and how I eat, my gut should feel better.*
-   *Blending helps digestion. The blender saves some of the work your intestines would need to do. Blending is also a cure for cancer-stress–related constipation. Think: smoothies smooth the stool passage! I sometimes call my smoothie "stool-ade."*

Switching to smoothies for many of my meals gave me good gut feelings. Twenty-four years later, five days a week, I still enjoy half of a freshly blended smoothie for breakfast (see recipe, pages 209–210), then sip on the rest for a mid-morning snack and often as a light lunch.

The sipping solution is one of the smartest solutions to the problems of healing from cancer, surgery, and chemo and radiation effects, and is even a tool for future cancer prevention. Over Dr. Bill's twenty-five years of healing from cancers and helping others heal, the sipping solution is the one simple tool that has gotten the greatest results and had the most lasting effects. Once you get used to enjoying the good gut feel and the steady mental and physical energy the sipping solution provides, you're also likely to continue this healthy eating habit for life.

Cancer Contributors	Benefits of the Sipping Solution
• Sugar spikes	• Sugar spikes less
• A diet low in antioxidants	• High in antioxidants
• A diet low in anti-cancer nutrients	• High in anti-cancer nutrients
	• Microbiome-friendly
• Microbiome upsets	• Lean-friendly
• Obesity and excess belly fat	• Smartens immune system
• A weakened immune system	

Blending is better than juicing. Like the Sears family, you probably have a couple old juicers in your garage that you have smartly replaced with high-speed blenders. The main reason that blending is better is that with juicing you throw away all the roughage and chewy stuff that your gut microbiome loves—the fiber. Although you don't digest the fiber, your microbiome uses it as fuel. It feeds on your leftovers! Also, keeping the fiber blunts the sugar spikes from juice. "Avoid sugar spikes" is one of the top anti-cancer lessons. Blending makes sense!

Dr. Bill notes: *During my rounds one day, I heard a blender going in a nearby hospital room. A nurse quipped: "Oh, that must be one of Dr. Sears's patients."*

Children healing from surgery or illnesses are especially fond of the sipping solution. As one of my little healing patients said, "I call my smoothie my soothie."

Smoothie-Making Tips

Make your smoothie *your* cancer-healing soothie. Enjoy our anti-cancer smoothie recipe on pages 209–210. A few tips for successful sipping:

Start low and go slow. The gut, an organ of habit, is likely to rebel with constipation or diarrhea if you drastically change your diet too fast. When first beginning the sipping solution, start with ingredients you know your gut already likes. Especially when healing from surgery or when starting gut-unfriendly chemotherapy, overwhelming your intestines with too many new ingredients all of a sudden is likely to literally give you a pain in the gut. Don't drink too much, too fast, at first either. Start with a few sips every hour or so and gradually increase the volume as your gut likes. Keep your smoothie cold in the fridge throughout the day or with an icepack.

Personalize your recipe. After a few weeks of taste-testing (learning to like less sweet foods) and gut-feeling many of the anti-cancer foods in our anti-cancer smoothie recipe on pages 209–210, you'll arrive at a personal healing recipe that your gut likes best. Of course, both your gut and your brain enjoy novelty, so you may want to periodically add or subtract a few foods.

Smart-fat your smoothie. The biggest mistake most shake-makers make is they don't include enough healthy fats. As you've learned, junk carbs make you fat, but healthy fats help keep you lean (see page 81). Another fat fact: fats increase the absorption of fat-soluble nutrients, such as vitamins A, D, E, and K, and anti-cancer antioxidants, such as carotenoids and flavonoids. Finally, fats give your smoothie a savory mouthfeel. The more you enjoy your anti-cancer smoothie, the longer you will continue to drink it. Makes sense! (See page 210 for a list of healthy fats.)

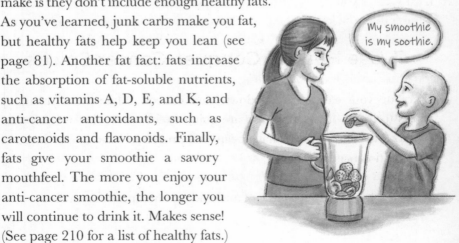

My smoothie is my soothie.

Savor Synergy

A healing term key to your healing diet is *synergy*, meaning the more diversity and color on your plate or in your bowl or blender, the more the conquer-cancer nutrients fight for you. Like a team of eleven players are more likely to score a touchdown than a team of only five, a multi-fruit and green vegetable smoothie or salad helps each food fight better against cancer than if you were to eat any one of those foods alone.

Make a Smart Choice!

Eating the Usual Cancer-Contributing Diet	Eating the Conquer-Cancer Diet
• Spikes blood sugar.	• Blunts blood sugar spikes.
• Stores belly fat.	• Leans out belly fat.
• Weakens immune system.	• Smartens immune system.
• Dulls healthy-eating decisions.	• Smartens eating decisions.

7. Use Healing Conquer-Cancer Spices

Spice up your eating to dial down your cancer! While there are many spices to help your healing, we are going to focus on what we call "the fabulous five," spices that have been well proven to have one or more of these anti-cancer effects:

- They're a rich source of antioxidant and anti-inflammatory nutrients.

- They have proven anti-cancer benefits both in humans and experimental animals.
- They help trigger apoptosis—the programmed death of cancer cells.
- They lessen adverse effects of cancer treatment and healing.

Turmeric Is a Terrific Conquer-Cancer Spice

Turmeric is a thoroughly researched spice proven especially healing for some of the common cancers: breast, colon, pancreatic, prostate, and lung. The list of proven anti-cancer effects of turmeric is impressive, in particular:

- It helps protect healthy cells from becoming cancerous.
- It lessens the growth of cancer cells.
- It helps make chemotherapy less toxic and more effective.

Turmeric tips:

- Keep a shaker of turmeric and a shaker of freshly ground pepper (which enhances turmeric's otherwise poor absorption) on your kitchen and dining tables.
- Grind your own turmeric from shavings of organic, dried turmeric roots.
- Strive for one full teaspoon each day. We sprinkle half a teaspoon of turmeric and black pepper on our omelets in the morning and on our salads in the evening.
- Partner turmeric with olive oil since this favorite anti-cancer oil improves the absorption of turmeric.
- Turmeric is especially flavorful when lightly heated in a hot salad (see Dr. Bill's hot salad, page 211).
- Capsules twice a day are fine if you don't like the taste of turmeric. Be sure the capsules also contain "piperine," the main anti-cancer ingredient in pepper (see below), to aid absorption.

> A teaspoon of turmeric and black pepper
> a day helps keep cancer away.

Enjoy Dr. Pepper

No, not the cola, but real ground black pepper. After learning that black pepper enhances the otherwise poor absorption of turmeric, a peppercorn-filled grinder became the centerpiece of our meals. Dr. Bill found he started craving pepper and even got a bit impatient when he couldn't find his pepper grinder. He wouldn't start a meal without it, as if our lone container of turmeric was missing its buddy.

Piperine, the main anti-cancer ingredient in pepper—think of it as "black gold"—is especially helpful in preventing colon cancer. The same mechanism that zings your taste buds and triggers a sneeze also triggers the pancreas to start producing digestive enzymes. It's as if the tongue tells the pancreas to start gearing up for what's coming down. Pepper also speeds up the time it takes food to move through your digestive tract and out, called "intestinal transit time." And as you already know, the less time undigested food products spend pressing against the lining of your colon, the less irritation to the lining and the less cancer. In laboratory studies on animals and humans, pepper has been shown to have anti-cancer effects not only on colon cancer, but on lung and breast cancers.

While piperine is found in all peppercorns, it is highest in black pepper, and it's best to grind the whole peppercorns as needed. Since marinating somewhat lessens the carcinogenic properties of meat, as you learned on page 100, try massaging ground black peppercorns into the meat as part of the marinade, especially on lamb loin—yum! And be sure to give those two tiny towers, the turmeric shaker and the peppercorn grinder, top honors when you dine.

"Curry Up" Your Cancer Healing

Back to that wisdom of the body you learned about on pages 16–17, during Dr. Bill's cancer healing he noticed a craving for more Indian foods. Indian curry uses a mixture of spices, such as turmeric, black pepper, and cumin seeds, that have anti-cancer effects. Could that be one of the reasons why Indians eating their traditional diet enjoy a much lower incidence of most cancers?

Garlic Is Great for Cancer Healing

We call garlic "the stink that heals." "Bill, you're reeking of garlic again," Martha would smilingly say. Spices get their aroma from the volatile oils they contain, and garlic is very "volatile." The "wow!" aroma you sniff from freshly crushed garlic, allicin, is the nutrient that ranks garlic along with turmeric as our top pick for science-supported healing spices.

"Garlic breath" was what first prompted Dr. Bill to research this potent medicinal spice. His logic: If you eat it and smell it on your breath and in your skin, you know it's reaching your lungs and being absorbed by your tissues. He found that garlic is a highly researched anti-cancer spice that helps lower the risk of nearly all major cancers, especially colon, liver, stomach, breast, brain, uterine, and lung. Besides many other anti-cancer effects, garlic helps block toxins from damaging DNA (reducing the chance of a healthy cell becoming cancerous), increases cell self-destruction (apoptosis), and—our favorite garlic anti-cancer effect—helps NK cells fight better against cancer cells.

To get the most medicinal effects from garlic, *crush* each clove in a garlic press shortly before eating. Newly crushed, raw garlic confers the most medicinal effects, but at the price of more garlic breath and skin reek. Cooking garlic can reduce its stinkiness, yet at the price of lessening some of its health effects.

We like to add freshly crushed raw garlic to sauces, guacamole, soups, marinades, and whatever other foods need spicing up. One of our favorite sauces is aioli, which is basically mayonnaise upgraded with garlic.

Martha's homemade pesto sauce features basil, olive oil, and garlic—triple yum! To get the most health effects from garlic while preserving his romance with his coauthor, Dr. Bill adds crushed garlic to his hot salad toward the end of its steaming. (See Dr. Bill's hot salad, page 211.) Martha uses garlic capsules instead. Look for "organic" on the label.

Cinnamon Is Yum-Yum!

After reading the research that cinnamon helps blunt sugar spikes (remember, blood sugar spikes feed cancer cells, as you learned on page 80), we now sprinkle cinnamon into our morning smoothies and on many of our desserts (such as muffins and pies), and for fun sometimes we put a cinnamon stick into our coffee or add a dash of ground cinnamon.

Ground cinnamon loses some of its fragrance, taste, and health properties over time, so replace it often. Spiceologists recommend buying Ceylon cinnamon online or at Indian markets. Cinnamon is also available in capsule form.

Ginger Is Good Against Cancer

Ginger may help relieve nausea from cancer therapy. Researchers at MD Anderson Cancer Center found that ginger can strengthen tumor-suppressor genes, the good guys in your genetic army that help keep genetic mutations from becoming cancerous. Dr. Bill grates organic ginger root into salads, soups, and smoothies. Martha prefers ginger powder in capsules.

Other healing herbs that merit honorable mention: rosemary, oregano, thyme, and mustard seeds.

---

8. Savor Science-Based Supplements (SBS)

During healing from cancer surgery, chemo, radiation therapy, and other cancer treatments, nutrition is often at a low, thanks to a combination of a weakened appetite, gastrointestinal upsets, and wound healing—just at the time when nutrition needs to be at its best. Science-based supplements help fill this gap. Note that the word "supplement" is just that—supplementation should be in addition to, and not instead of, eating the anti-cancer foods listed on page 84.

Supplements can be confusing, and your passion to heal and your drive to take anything that may help can make you vulnerable to marketing over science. To help guide you through the maze of nutritional supplements and choose those that best fit you, keep in mind the following three rules:

1. Do I need it but don't eat it, therefore I must take it?
2. Show me the science.
3. Show me the source.

Below, we've outlined our four favorite science-based supplements to support cancer healing and overall immune system health:

Top Cancer Contributors	How Science-Based Supplements May Help
• Weakened immune system	• Support your immune system
• Inflammation	• Lessen inflammation
• Oxidation	• Provide antioxidants
• Stress imbalance	• Help calm stress
• Microbiome imbalance	• Feed your microbiome

Oh My Omegas!

See pages 86–89 for why seafood-based omega-3s are our top choice of anti-cancer nutrients.

If you're not fond of fish or fish oil, or if you're a vegetarian, you may need to take a vegan-based seafood source of omega-3s, a supplement sourced from sea *algae*. In one study, people who ate an algae source of omega-3s enjoyed greater fighting ability of their NK cells. See AskDrSears.com /omega-3supplements for the sea plant–based omega-3s we recommend.

Note to vegans: Seed sources of omega-3s, such as flaxseed and chia seeds, are not as biologically active as sea plant sources. If you are a vegan, we recommend measuring your omegas (see how, page 89) to see if your current diet gives you a sufficient level of omega-3s or if you need to take a sea plant source of omega-3s as a supplement. In our experience, most vegans need to take at least 1,000 milligrams of omega-3 DHA/EPA per day to reach the 8 percent level needed for sufficient cellular health.

Vitamin D Can Decrease Cancer

Back to our original mantra for selecting science-based supplements: Do you need it? You are at high risk of insufficient blood levels of vitamin D if you:

- Infrequently spend time in nature.
- Are over sixty years old.
- Live in a northern latitude.
- Suffer from an immune-deficiency illness.
- Are depressed (vitamin D also wears the hat of an antidepressant).
- Are obese (in people with obesity, vitamin D is trapped in excess fat instead of reaching cells throughout the body).
- Eat insufficient amounts of vitamin D–rich foods like wild salmon and egg yolk.

Recent studies reveal that nearly 90 percent of U.S. adults have a vitamin D level below the optimal range of 40 to 60 ng/ml.

Senior Alert!

As we age, we need more vitamin D. Most of our vitamin D comes from sun exposure turning cholesterol into vitamin D, and the older we get, the less cholesterol we have in our skin. Researchers found that seventy-year-olds make 70 percent less vitamin D from

---

sun exposure than twenty-year-olds. Also, vitamin D insufficiency is associated with an increased incidence of breast, prostate, and colon cancers, the most common cancers seniors get.

How vitamin D helps defeat cancer. Vitamin D is just what the cancer doctor ordered!

To prevent and heal from cancer you mainly need:

- *A smarter brain.* Vitamin D is a "neuroprotectant." Neurons are rich with vitamin D *receptors*, telling vitamin D, "Come on in, we need you." (Perhaps this is why vitamin D is dubbed an anti-*D*-pressant.)
- *A smarter immune system.* Sufficient blood levels of vitamin D strengthen the immune system—and a weakened immune system is one of the top contributors to cancer. The relationship between vitamin D and immune system health was recently highlighted by a study showing that patients infected with the COVID-19 virus got less sick and improved faster the higher their blood level of vitamin D.
- *Better blood vessels.* Better blood supply, better healing. Vitamin D helps relax the usual arterial stiffness that occurs with aging.

Vitamin D also acts as a cancer-suppressant by reducing the growth and aggressiveness of cancer cells, telling cells to "Cool it, and don't become an aggressive, renegade cancer cell!"

To be sure you are vitamin-D sufficient, have your blood level checked. If the result is below 40 ng/ml, you will need to eat more vitamin D–rich foods (6 ounces of wild Pacific salmon contains 2,000 IU of vitamin D) and most likely take a vitamin D3 supplement of between 1,000 and 2,000 units per day. Then recheck your blood level in two to three months.

To learn more about vitamin D—why you need it, how to test it, and how much to take—see AskDrSears.com/vitamin-D.

Women, Read This!

A 2018 study from the GrassrootsHealth Nutrient Research Institute showed that women over the age of fifty-five who enjoyed a vitamin D level of 60 ng/ml or greater had an 80 percent reduced risk of breast cancer compared with those whose vitamin D level was 20 ng/ml or less. A previous study from 2014 at the University of California San Diego School of Medicine showed that the average vitamin D level of patients with breast cancer in the United States was 17 ng/ml.

Plant-Food Extracts Help Fill Nutritional Gaps

Here is another area where the rule "If you don't eat it but need it, you must take it" really shines. Amid all the confusion about what the best anti-cancer foods are, there is one simple conclusion on which all trusted cancer-care providers agree: the more vegetables (especially leafy *greens*) and other plant-based foods you eat, the lower your risk. (This is especially true of cancer, but also of just about every disease you don't want to get.) Plant-based foods shine both as cancer-preventers and cancer-healers, as they support tissue healing when you do get sick.

Naturally, you're wondering how much plant food you need to eat each day to help your healing and lower your risk of future disease. Answer: at least ten (fist-size) servings a day. We had to go through this thought process, and you probably will, too: "I may not like all those veggies, but I also don't like cancer. Therefore, I will learn to like eating more vegetables."

After learning this, we changed our daily diet. We now sip on multi-fruit and veggie smoothies in the morning (see our conquer-cancer smoothie recipe, pages 209–210) and chew on multi-veggie salads in the evening (see our conquer-cancer salad, page 211). But because there are days when we still may not be able to eat the desired ten-plus servings of fruits and veggies, we also take several science-based fruit and vegetable supplements.

Dr. Bill's favorite plant-food supplements. *Early on in my cancer-healing journey, I researched science-based supplements that would give us extracts of many plant-based foods, especially fruits and vegetables, to help fill any gaps in our diet. The one I found that was supported by the most research was Juice Plus+ Fruit, Vegetable, and Berry Blend capsules, which include extracts of over thirty-one plant-based foods. Twenty years later I am still taking the trio. (See references on the scientific studies of Juice Plus+ plant-based supplements at JuicePlus.com /clinicalresearch.)*

Astaxanthin Is Awesome

Astaxanthin is Mother Nature's most powerful antioxidant, and the carotenoid nutrient that makes our top anti-cancer food, salmon, pink. (Carotenoids are the deeply colored antioxidants in many plant foods.) Carotenoids are "color-full," and colorful foods fight cancer. And remember, the deeper the color, usually the more anti-cancer nutrients.

Dr. Bill's astaxanthin trip to Hawaii. *When I first started reading the science behind astaxanthin, I was driven to learn more about this pink powerhouse. My homework led me to visit the Big Island of Hawaii, where the source of some of the world's best astaxanthin is grown in ponds, to meet biochemist Dr. Gerald Cysewski, who pioneered astaxanthin awareness and how to grow it. From him, I learned that Hawaiian astaxanthin is a concentrated extract from sea plants. By this time, I had already learned that extracted seafoods are top conquer-cancer foods. While humans have managed to mess up the soil and weaken its nutrient richness, Mother Nature still protects her aquatic sources.*

Science supports that astaxanthin supplements have these conquer-cancer abilities:

- Smarten the immune system by increasing the fighting abilities of cancer-fighting NK cells.
- Help protect DNA from damage that causes cells to become cancerous.
- Lessen oxidation and inflammation, two top cancer contributors.

In laboratory studies, astaxanthin has also been shown to slow the growth of tumor cells. And there are many studies showing that people whose diets are high in astaxanthin's carotenoid cousin, beta carotene, show a reduced incidence of cancers. (To learn more about Hawaiian astaxanthin, see Dr. Bill's book *Natural Astaxanthin: Hawaii's Supernutrient*.)

Spirulina Is a Star Seafood Supplement

Meet Hawaiian spirulina, a nutrient-rich, easily digestible vegetable from microalgae that, like Hawaiian astaxanthin, is grown in freshwater ponds. It is mostly protein, around 60 percent, and is richer in the powerful antioxidant beta carotene than any other fruit or vegetable. It's also rich in many other nutrients that people with cancer are deficient in, including iron, beta carotene, zeaxanthin, B-vitamins, vitamins K1 and K2, and more.

For updates on science-based nutritional supplements, see AskDrSears.com/supplements.

Dr. Bill's Daily Conquer-Cancer Diet

Cancer caused me to change my eating habits for good. Here's a summary of my diet:

- I begin the day with my "sipping solution"—a conquer-cancer smoothie (see page 209). On non-smoothie days, I eat a multi-veggie omelet with guacamole.
- I sip on green tea with lemon throughout the day. (Swishing with green tea also helps dental health; see the oral health–cancer connection, page 207.)
- For dinner, I eat a large conquer-cancer salad (see page 211), often topped with a 6-ounce fillet of wild salmon.
- I graze by my "rule of twos" (see page 98).

- I snack on eggs, homemade trail mix, and organic apple slices with nut butter.
- I aim to eat wild seafood three to four times a week, and wild game (especially venison or grass-fed and grass-finished lamb or beef) for dinner two to three times a month.
- I have one glass of organic red wine two evenings a week, sipped slowly with dinner.
- For an occasional treat, I enjoy *homemade* muffins, apple/raisin pie, and homemade ice cream.
- I take several daily supplements:
  - *Omega-3s:* enough to keep my omega-3 index above 8 percent.
  - *Vitamin D3:* 2,000 IU daily, enough to keep my level above 50 ng/ml.
  - *Juice Plus+* fruit, vegetable, and berry capsules to add antioxidants.
  - *Spirulina*, often added to my smoothie.
- While I don't often count calories, I aim to eat 2,000 to 2,200 calories and burn 2,500 to 2,700 calories (see "Burn More Than You Eat," page 101).

Dr. Bill's daily conquer-cancer diet made memorable. In short, you want to be known as a:

- Smoothie sipper
- Nut nibbler
- Green tea swisher
- Smart sea-foodie
- Good grazer
- Smart snacker
- Salad sampler

- Long chewer
- Carb cutter
- Science-based supplement taker

Conquer-cancer   green tea   nibble on nuts   Conquer-cancer   treat
smoothie   and eggs   salad

Conquer-cancer Plate

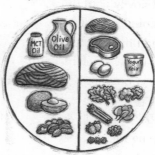

45-50%
healthy
fats

25-30%
protein

25-30%
carbs

The Leaner You Are, the Less Cancer You Are Likely to Get

The best "medicine" you can take to heal from cancer and to prevent future cancer from developing?

> Stay lean!

"Lean" is the top cancer-healing and cancer-prevention word in your growing conquer-cancer vocabulary. Lean does not mean "skinny." It means having the muscle mass and percentage of body fat that is right for your individual body type.

There are five main reasons why staying lean helps you heal from cancer:

1. Carcinogens are stored in excess fat tissue.
2. Excess body fat raises blood sugar levels, a top cancer-feeder.
3. Excess fat can weaken your immune system.
4. Excess fat can cause hormone imbalances.

5. Excess belly fat is pro-inflammatory, and inflammation fuels cancer.

Besides the statistical studies listing excess belly fat as the top cancer contributor, another reason that motivated Dr. Bill to move more, sit less, and reduce his belt size was the scientific finding by cancer researchers that excess fat, especially belly fat, is the principal storage site of carcinogens from both the food we eat and the air we breathe—hence the label "toxic waist."

You already know about the effect of high blood sugar levels and a weakened immune system on cancer growth. But out-of-balance hormones are a risk factor, too. Extra body fat—and again, especially belly fat—increases blood levels of estrogen in both men and women. *Fat cells make estrogen.* Certain cancers, especially breast and uterine cancers, are fueled by high levels of estrogen.

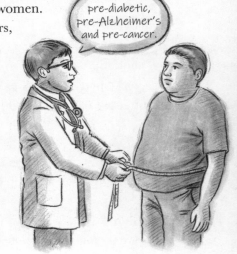

You're pre-diabetic, pre-Alzheimer's and pre-cancer.

Another staggering statistic that caused us to stay on our L.E.A.N. family path was in our medical practice, as well as in the pediatric literature: young adults today have the highest incidence of cancer at any time in human history. They're also the fattest at any time in human history. Any correlation? The science suggests yes.

Fat Loss Over Weight Loss

Waist-size reduction is much more cancer-preventing and healing than *weight loss*. In fact, putting on extra muscle weight (muscle weighs more than fat) while losing belly fat is good for you. More muscle, less sugar-spiking.

Since the incidence of nearly all cancers increases as the extra fat around your middle increases, the top tools to help you stay lean are eating our conquer-cancer diet and moving more and sitting less—which you will learn how to do in our next chapter.

Why Cancer Increases with Age—If You Let It!

Once upon a time, cancer was one of those "age-related" diseases. While today it is becoming an epidemic of all ages, there are several reasons why the older you get, the more at risk you are:

- As you learned on page 5, cancer occurs due to what we call a *cumulative effect:* it is the result of small doses of carcinogens that accumulate over a period of time. For example, every day that you eat a little bit of nonorganic, heavily sprayed food, you get a little bit more pesticides in your cells. Over years and years, these toxins gradually reach higher and higher levels in more cells, and your healthy cells begin to become cancerous.
- We provide more grow-food for cancer as we age. Our sugar metabolism gets quirkier as we get older; carbs spike more and insulin levels rise.
- Aging cells produce fewer of their own cell-protecting antioxidants.
- We usually accumulate more belly fat as we age. Since toxins are stored in fat, the more belly fat you have, the more carcinogens you accumulate. Belly fat also contributes to bigger sugar spikes.
- We lose muscle mass as we age. Muscle helps blunt sugar spikes. Less muscle, more fat, leads to more cancer-feeding sugar spikes.
- Our immune system, including our naturally protective anti-cancer cellular machinery, gets "old," too. The

gradual weakening of the immune system as we age may be partially responsible for the associated increase in cancer.

- Seniors often sleep less and make less of the sleep-promoting and cancer-conquering hormone melatonin.

In addition, with many cancers, it can take years for the cancer cells to truly misbehave. You may "get cancer" early, but not feel cancer because the organ isn't damaged enough yet. (Hopefully, someday there will be a blood test for early cancer markers so that you can detect it before you feel it.)

Also worth noting: Not only does the risk of getting cancer increase with age, so do the adverse effects of cancer therapies.

Our conclusion? The older you are, the smarter you need to be about preventing cancer. Keep your immune system young and healthy by eating smart; moving more, sitting less; and meditating more, agitating less. (We discuss these top three stay-young habits even more thoroughly in our partner book, *The Dr. Sears T5 Wellness Plan*.)

The double-good news is that the tools that help you heal from cancer are the same ones that will help you live longer. In fact, you may find it more positive to think of them as "my longevity recipe" than as cancer-healing tools.

Chapter 6

. . . .

Move More, Sit Less, Heal Better

C ancer researchers have shown that the risk of nearly all cancers goes down the more your daily movement goes up.

This makes sense. Exercise—like eating the anti-cancer way—lowers your biochemical cancer feeders: IGF-1 levels and blood sugar spikes. "The sitting disease" is one of the newest illnesses in the doctor's dictionary, and one of the most preventable causes of cancer. Remember this mantra:

> The leaner, the less cancer.

To refresh your memory, cancer healing requires three main things:

1. Smartening your conquer-cancer army to fight better for you.
2. Making the environment in your cellular garden (see page 25) feed healthy cells and fight cancer cells.
3. Reducing cancer-cell fertilizers.

Movement does all three.

Better blood flow, better health. Every organ of your body is only as healthy as the quality and quantity of blood flow to it. Movement makes *more blood flow* to all the vital organs throughout your body.

Better blood flow, better health.

Why Movers Heal Better Than Sitters

Move More	Sit More
• Smarter conquer-cancer army	• Weaker conquer-cancer army inside
• Fewer blood-sugar spikes	• More blood-sugar spikes
• Leaner waist	• Fatter, cancer-feeding waist
• Fewer cancer fertilizers stored	• Cancer fertilizers stored in body fat
• Less inflammation	• More "-itis" illnesses
• Smarter conquer-cancer mindset	• Weaker conquer-cancer mindset
• More optimistic	• Possibly more pessimistic

Sit and stew is bad for you!

Movement Mobilizes Your Conquer-Cancer Army

Get ready to say "Wow!" The natural killer cells of regular exercisers, whom we call "movers," have higher levels and better fighting ability than those of sitters. One theory as to how exercise helps fight cancer is that movement causes your muscles to contract, squeezing blood and lymphatic vessels, which makes blood and lymph flow faster. This can help your NK cells and other white blood cells in your immune system army patrol more of the body faster, and with more soldiers.

Besides directly mobilizing the immune system, movement mobilizes belly fat (as you learned on page 122), which helps shrink your waist. Shrink your "toxic waist," shrink your cancer.

Next time you're running, swimming, taking a brisk walk, dancing, or doing any other vigorous movement, think: "I'm mobilizing my anti-cancer army. I'm making my NK cells fight smarter. I'm shrinking my toxic waist."

Cancer cells can become smarter than your own NK cells—if you allow it. Part of the adaptation cancer cells go through as they replicate is learning to avoid being detected by NK cells. They also learn how to grab on to more growth factors in their environment to help them grow and multiply. That's why helping smarten your NK cell army so it can better fight the always-learning opposing cancer-cell invaders is so important. (See more about how movement mobilizes NK cells in Chapter 2, page 36.)

Movement Blunts Sugar Spikes

Follow this logic: Cancer cells feed on sugar spikes. Exercise blunts sugar spikes. This is another reason why movers are likely to heal better from cancer than sitters.

Movement blunts spikes because *exercise increases insulin sensitivity*. It opens the doors to cells that let in blood sugar, so that more sugar gets used up by healthy cells and less is left over to feed the cancer cells. Insulin *in*sensitivity, also called "pre-diabetes" and "type 2 diabetes," is now the top medical disease in America and throughout much of the world, making too many of us not just "pre-diabetes" but also "pre-cancer."

Exercise Improves Every Organ

Exercise lessens "comorbidities," doctor-speak for other illnesses present before and during your cancer. Nearly every organ in your body enjoys better health the more you move: brain, gut, heart, bone, immune system, and more.

Exercise Goes to Your Head

Becoming a wise partner in your own cancer healing requires you to be cancer-smart. You will need to make wise decisions and remember many things, such as taking daily chemo medicine, what medical questions to ask at your doctor's appointments, and more. Movement increases blood flow to your brain, which helps repair brain tissue and keep it healthy. Also, movement pumps into your brain a natural brain-growth fertilizer (BGF) to help you grow the new brain tissue you'll need during your healing.

You may notice that many of our conquer-cancer tools highlight the brain, especially movement. In Chapter 1 you learned why: your brain is the commander-in-chief of your conquer-cancer army inside. More movement, more blood flow to your brain; smarter brain, smarter cancer-recovery decisions. You can feel that!

Throughout your cancer-healing journey, you will also need to cope with toxic thoughts that pollute your mind and slow your healing, such as: "Is my cancer going away?" "How will this new chemo drug affect me?" "Will my cancer come back?" These are normal and usual worries, but they can infect your mind if you let them. Exercise helps! During exercise, toxic thoughts usually lessen or go away before they have a chance to be stored deeper in your brain and become chronic.

Movers became shakers. A study from the University of Miami revealed that when compared with sitters, movers were better able to shake off "bad news." Exercisers seem to be able to get negative thoughts to "run away" more quickly, so they don't settle in.

Movement Balances Your Hormones

Back to our earlier teaching: cancer healing is about putting your body back into biochemical, hormonal, and metabolic balance. The growth of estrogen-dependent cancers, such as breast, ovarian, and uterine cancers, can be increased by excess estrogen levels. Similarly, increased testosterone levels can increase prostate and testicular cancer growth. Exercise balances these hormones for the hormonal health you need.

Beat Breast Cancer Alert!

Science shows that women who exercise the most get breast cancer the least. This "exercise effect" is more cancer-preventative ᵗhe greater the duration and intensity of the movements.

How to Open Your Own Personal Conquer-Cancer Pharmacy: A Doctor–Patient Conversation

You have inside your body your own personal pharmacy that can make medicines to help your cancer heal. These medicines have a triple-good effect: they help you heal from cancer, they help lessen the adverse effects of treatment, and many of them help conventional treatments work better. The key to opening this pharmacy? Movement!

Imagine a conversation between an oncologist, Dr. Self-Help, and her patient (oops . . . partner in healing!) Susan:

"Before we discuss the treatment that I believe is best for your cancer, such as options of surgery, chemotherapy, and radiation therapy, I want you to know that you also have your own conquer-cancer army inside that can help kill your cancer cells. I'm going to share with you things you can do to prepare your army to fight better for you."

(The doctor discusses the natural killer cells, similar to what we present on pages 30–34.)

"Also, Susan, in addition to your immune-system army inside, your body is blessed with its own personal conquer-cancer pharmacy. Pay close attention, because what I'm about to teach you won the Nobel Prize."

(Naturally, the patient's interest is piqued.)

"Let me ask you a question, Susan. If you were designing the greatest machine ever made—the human body—yet you knew we humans were going to mess it up by how we eat, think, and live, wouldn't you want to put inside your body a pharmacy that stocks and dispenses medicines to help fight disease? That's exactly what we have.

"Yes, I can prescribe some healing medicines, and I will when needed, but the medicines your body makes are better than the medicines you take because they're custom-made just for you. They come out at the right time, in the right dose, and they don't have any adverse effects. Unfortunately, many of the medicines I can prescribe for you do have adverse effects."

Susan is riveted. "So, doctor, I actually have my own personalized pharmacy inside that can make medicines that help me heal?"

"Yes, you do, but you've got to take care of that pharmacy, to help it make the best medicines for you," the doctor replies.

"Okay, I can't wait—tell me how," Susan replies.

"Here's a picture of your blood vessel. Notice the lining, called the endothelium. This is where your pharmacy is. What a smart design! If you wanted medicines to get into your bloodstream as quickly as possible, the lining of the blood vessels is where you'd put them."

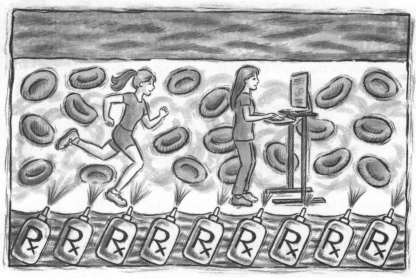

Mandi the Mover

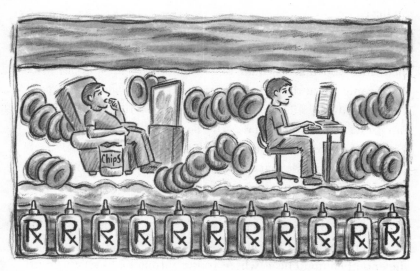

Sam the Sitter

"That makes sense!" says Susan.

"Notice the microscopic medicine bottles. You have trillions of them. And the medicines inside these medicine bottles are gas, not liquid, so they dissolve quicker. Picture these trillions of little squirt bottles pumping medicines into your blood."

Another "Wow!" from Susan.

"There are two things you need to do to stock your pharmacy, open it, and help it make better medicines for you."

"What are those two things?" Susan asks.

"Very simply, eat smart—and move more," Dr. Self-Help says. "Consider Mandi the Mover. When she moves, her blood flows faster over the top of the medicine bottles. Movement creates a shear force that opens the medicine bottles and releases her natural medicines. That's why 'move more, sit less' is one of my top prescriptions for you.

"Mandi also keeps 'sticky stuff'—sticky, sugary, processed fake foods—out of her mouth, to keep sticky stuff out of her blood and off the lining of her blood vessels, so it doesn't clog the squirt bottles.

"Now, consider Sam the Sitter. He does the opposite. He sits too much and puts too much sticky stuff in his mouth. As a result, his medicine bottles don't open.

"Susan, to help yourself heal, which one of these people do you want to model—Sam the Sitter or Mandi the Mover?"

Susan says, "Obviously, Mandi the Mover. Doctor, I am now motivated to do this. Of course, I've heard all about how diet and exercise is good for you, but now that I know why and what's going on in my body, I'm now more committed to making a change."

"And Susan, as an added incentive, science shows that many of the tools we're going to talk about in our sessions, including moving more, also help the medicines I'm going to prescribe for you work better."

"That's doubly good! I like that. Thank you, Doctor!" Susan says.

For a riveting watch, don't miss our video on your endothelial pharmacy at youtube.com/watch?v=1fVzxsVJ7vA.

View It and Do It

For a motivating thirty-minute video of Dr. Bill in action, see "9 Simple Steps to Prime-Time Health" at vimeo.com/11272800.

Guy Alert: Movement Modulates Male Menopause

Andropause, or male menopause, is a drop in testosterone—the natural male muscle-builder—that occurs in men in middle age. Weaker muscle contributes to higher blood sugar—a top cancer-feeder. Add the pot belly that often also accompanies male menopause and you have a double whammy set up for cancer. Prescription: The older you get, the more muscle-strengthening exercises you need to do.

> Better blood flow, better thinking! Better blood flow, better healing! Movement does both.

How to Make Your Movements Match Your Healing

Whatever exercises increase your blood flow (recognized by an increased heart rate and breathing rate) are healing. If you're recovering from surgery or other medical treatments (such as in-dwelling catheters) that temporarily prevent you from strenuous exercise, swimming, or brisk walking, try:

- Moving your arms and/or legs with light weights attached.
- Enjoying *isometrics*: holding flexed muscles tight until you "feel the burn!"
  - *While sitting*, raise your thighs, cross your lower legs and hold for twenty to thirty seconds, while pressing your ankles together. Next, flex your arms and biceps and hold until you feel the effort in your muscles. Then, push your palms together while flexing your arm muscles and pecs to continue that feeling a bit longer.
  - *While standing*, flex your knees slightly; flex your thighs and glute muscles and hold. Repeat while slightly on tiptoe.

With isometrics, even though you're just flexing your muscles, you are still increasing the healing blood flow through your body. For isometrics in action, see AskDrSears.com/isometrics and our partner book, *The Dr. Sears T5 Wellness Plan.*

Go Outside and Play—Chase Cancer Away!

Remember wise Dr. Mom's prescription to "Go outside and play"? This simple "medicine" can help heal cancer.

Dr. Bill notes: *Oftentimes, I begin a conquer-cancer consultation with the question: "How many minutes each day do you spend moving in nature?" The higher your dosage of nature-therapy medicine, the more likely you are to heal.*

The benefits of forest bathing. After a long and mentally exhausting lecture day at a medical and parenting conference in Japan, Dr. Bill's hosts announced, "We're going to take you and Mrs. Sears out for some *shinrin-yoku.*" We thought this might be a Japanese drink, so we were surprised when Mr. Sakinishi drove us to a pine forest, his "happy place,"

Healing Effects of Movement Outdoors

- Lowers stress
- Lessens pain
- Lessens inflammation
- Increases overall sense of well-being

- Lifts depression
- Lowers anxiety
- Increases number of NK cells and their fighting ability

Very few medications can show all these effects!

to enjoy an hour of "forest bathing," after which we felt a deep sense of mental and physical peace.

Researchers from the Japanese Society of Forest Medicine at Nippon Medical School have studied the physiologic effects of forest bathing by wiring up volunteers with sensors to measure what was going on in their brains during their walk in the woods. They also took various blood and saliva measurements before and after their forest-bathing medicine. The researchers discovered that stress hormones went down; happy hormones went up; heart rate and blood pressure were healthier; and, take note, *their levels of natural killer cells*—the Navy Seals of your conquer-cancer army inside—went up. They also found that blood levels of the cancer-killing bullets that NK cells shoot into cancer cells, called perforins (think "perforate"), went up in the forest bathers. Wow! Anything that smartens NK cells to fighting cancer, bring it on!

Studies show that even a day of forest bathing can improve the fighting ability of NK cells for a week. Simply put, time in nature puts the body-mind back into balance, and a balanced body-mind helps healing.

Dr. Bill's "vitamin G" story. *During my first cancer-healing, I kept careful records of any correlation between what I did and how I felt. Spending much of the day outside in natural sunlight and around greenery—even better, spending most of my movement or exercise time outdoors—made me feel so much physically and emotionally better, especially when coping with the side effects of the chemo and* *radiation. The more I surrounded myself with "greenspace"–the higher my dose of "vitamin G"–the better I healed.*

Giving in to my doctor's mindset of "show me the science" and the internal "why" behind what I felt led me to consult Dr. Eva Selhub, a Japanese neurologist, instructor of medicine at Harvard Medical School, and author of Your Brain on Nature. *Dr. Selhub summarized my cravings for movement in nature: "Movement in nature is exercise squared!"*

Greenspace movement promotes green peace. That healing "something in the air" is the vapors of nature, called volatile oils—the "medicine" plants make to protect their own health. These have been shown to enhance production of the brain's own calming chemical, gamma-aminobutyric acid (GABA), in addition to boosting serotonin. Since mental stress of dwelling on negative thoughts can partially sabotage some of the healthful effects of exercise, and positive and peaceful thoughts are more likely to overshadow negative ones while outside, this may explain why movement in nature is also called "medicine for the mind."

In one fascinating study, Japanese researchers infused vaporized volatile oils from cypress trees into a roomful of volunteers and found their stress hormone levels went down (and their NK cell activity went up) on the days they breathed this healing air compared to the days they didn't.

> To chase toxic thoughts away, go outside and play.

Designing Your Own Home Greenspace

Suppose medical or environmental conditions prevent you from a daily brisk walk in the woods or park. With a bit of ingenuity, you may be able to duplicate your own greenspace indoors. While movement in nature is healing, just being in or next to nature can also heal for two reasons: what you see, and what you smell.

Because the eyes are the windows to your brain and your brain is the commander of your immune system, what is pleasing to the eye is pleasing to the brain and to your immune system. Consult a house-plant expert near you to safely personalize your greenspace rooms, especially your office and bedroom.

Dr. Bill prescribes:
Take a deep breath in greenspace.

Vitamin G and Vitamin D:
Partners in Cancer Healing

As you learned on pages 113–114, those with higher vitamin D blood levels:

- Have a healthier immune system.
- Have a lower risk of and better healing from breast cancer.

The medicines your body makes by moving in nature (greenspace, or vitamin G) and the vitamin D the sunshine helps your body make are partners in health.

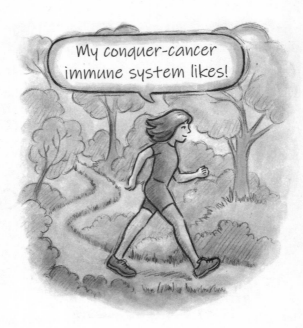

If you were to ask us to summarize our conquer-cancer plan in one simple sentence, we would say:

> Believe you will heal; eat more fruits, vegetables, and seafood; and go outside and play.

In this chapter you learned a vital lesson in total-body health: better blood flow, better health. Carrying on with this self-help theme in the next chapter, we add: the more peaceful thoughts flow, the better cancer-healing armies grow. Read on!

Chapter 7

· · · · · · · · · · · · · · · · · · ·

Peace Be with You

W hen we asked a friend who healed from cancer how she stayed calm and peaceful during her healing journey, she smiled and said, "I'm my own CEO—chief emotional operator."

Cancer is a *dis-ease*. Stress management—or the term we prefer, "mind management"—brings you peace. We notice that one characteristic of people who better handle dealing with cancer is *they learn mind-management strategies*. This helps them become less fearful and more focused on finding meaning and purpose in life. They also believe more deeply that they will heal (see related section on the "belief effect," on pages 12 and 34).

We don't want you to think "stress causes cancer" because there is little science to support that. Yet science shows that stress *can* sabotage your healing. That's why the conquer-cancer mindset and belief effect that we began this book with are so important.

The admonition "Don't stress" is impossible for most of us. It's also not biologically correct. Better advice is "Balance your stress." A fascinating new field called *psycho-oncology* is revealing how prolonged, unresolved stress can increase your risk of getting cancer and decrease your chances of healing from cancer.

Two main reasons a healthy cell turns cancerous are: 1) the tissue environment in which the cell lives (the garden the cell grows in, as we explain on page 25, or your L.E.A.N.—lifestyle, exercise, attitude, and nutrition) is unhealthy, and 2) your conquer-cancer army inside becomes too weak to destroy newly cancerous cells before they can grow and spread. As we'll see in this chapter, prolonged, unresolved stress affects both of these.

Science Says: Manage Your Mind, Manage Your Cancer

People who master mind management:

- Become more positive—positivity promotes longevity.
- Have a less cluttered mind, enabling them to stick with their conquer-cancer program.
- Sleep better (see Chapter 8, "Sleep Cancer Away").
- Enjoy a smarter conquer-cancer army inside.
- Suffer fewer blood-sugar spikes—a top cancer-fertilizer.
- Handle the adverse effects of chemotherapy better.
- Make smarter health decisions to fight their cancer.

Imagine top cancer scientists being asked to vote on what they believe—and science supports—to be top beat-cancer tips. A big winner: *Manage your mind, manage your cancer.*

Martha's mind change: *I remember very well how my cancer-treatment team helped me put aside thoughts and worries that were not at all useful (for example, "I should have known sooner"). My medical oncologist reframed my thinking to let go of that "if only" and "what if" inner prompting so I could see things in a better light, focus on the here and now, and begin to move forward. I got similar support from my surgeon and even my radiation oncologist, who showed me a path through the rigors of my radiation protocol—"We will beat this together!"*

How Mind Management
Helps Cancer Healing

Stress Is a Cancer-Cell Fertilizer

It's those hormones again! Stress hormones—namely the big one, cortisol—increase blood-sugar spikes. Remember:

> Stress increases blood sugar; sugar feeds cancer.

Mind Management Supports Your Anti-Cancer Army

Get ready to say "Wow!" Prolonged levels of high stress hormones can greatly decrease the fighting ability of your conquer-cancer army—especially your NK cells.

A fascinating piece of cancer detective work that further motivated us to upgrade our stress management was the discovery that NK cells have stress hormone receptors. Worrisome thoughts create electrochemical vibrations, and the receptor "doors" on the NK cells feel these vibrations. These negative vibes "stress out" NK cells, which weakens their ability to fight cancer cells.

Molecules of emotion—cancer-preventing *and* cancer-causing. One of our favorite neuroscientists, Dr. Candace Pert, discovered in her "vibes" research that some of the top stress hormones, such as norepinephrine and cortisol, in appropriate doses can boost quick and creative thinking, which can help you make the kind of smart decisions that let you personalize, and be a partner in, your cancer-treatment plan. Dr. Pert calls these cellular influencers "molecules of emotion."

In the right doses, and at the right times, these molecules of emotion can help keep healthy cells from turning cancerous and already cancerous cells from growing. If, however, your stress hormones are too high for too long, they can sabotage your healing.

Positivity smartens NK cells. A fascinating study by neuroscientist Dr. Richard Davidson, founder and director of the Center for Healthy Minds at the University of Wisconsin–Madison, found that optimists enjoy two cancer-healing perks: a higher level of circulating NK cells, and NK cells that are less impaired by stress.

Stress Sabotages Sleep

Many people who are stressed out during the day have difficulty sleeping at night, and poor-quality sleep can harm cancer healing in two ways: First, it causes hormonal imbalance the next day by decreasing your levels of leptin, the "eat less" hormone, and increasing the levels of ghrelin, the "eat more" hormone. This becomes a recipe for excess body fat, especially if your "eat more" prompt means eating more cancer-fertilizing fake foods; as we learned on pages 121–122, excess body fat in itself can become a cancer fertilizer. Second, poor quality sleep can increase the level of stress hormones circulating in your body both at night and the next day.

In addition, the sleep hormone, melatonin, is itself a natural anti-cancer antioxidant. Less quality sleep means less melatonin (see page 151).

Stress Causes Adrenal Fatigue

Many of your stress hormones are made in your adrenal glands. If you are always "on edge" and your adrenal glands are constantly in overdrive from producing these hormones, they can wear out. This results in something called adrenal fatigue, which can further sabotage your cancer-healing by sapping your energy and your motivation to help yourself heal. This high-stress hormone cascade also can dampen thyroid hormone production, which can make you more tired.

People with cancer are often already battling feelings of hopelessness and helplessness. Don't waste your energy wearing out your adrenals; save that energy to keep your mind focused on healing.

"Don't be a victim." This phrase jumped out at Martha when she was skimming through the booklet she received from her breast cancer oncology team. These four words alone helped her steer clear of that thought pathway and gave her important direction right at the beginning of her treatment, even before she had her surgery.

> When you feel well, you heal well!

Cancer healing is total-body healing. Yes, your brain and immune system are the top cancer fighters, yet all your other hormone-producing organs also play their part. A cancer-healing body is one that is operating in "hormonal harmony."

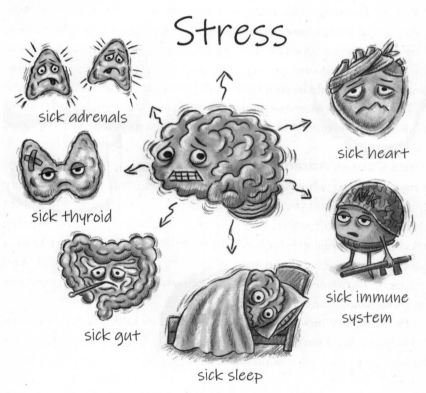

Stress

sick adrenals

sick heart

sick thyroid

sick immune system

sick gut

sick sleep

The Top Conquer-Cancer
Stress-Management Tools

Replace Toxic Thoughts with Happy Thoughts

Trash toxic thoughts! Take inventory and purge yourself of people, places, and thoughts that grow your worry center. People healing from cancer need a bigger happy center and bigger toxic-thoughts trash bin in their brain.

Save your energy for thinking about what you can do to help yourself heal—something over which you have control. Don't waste it worrying about things you can't control!

Mantras are mind-balancing. For us, "mantra" means "mind prompt." Fill your mind with cancer-conquering prompts: short catchphrase "reminders" that inspire you to replay a scene, song, or event that quiets your mind and puts you in a peaceful state. Picture the effect of these mantras on your new conquer-cancer mind in the same way that the photo on the wallpaper of your cellphone that makes you smile every time you pick it up.

Read More About How to Have a Happy Brain

For a science-based and easy-to-understand plan to trash toxic thoughts, plus further empower and equip your own personal stress-management toolbox, see *The Healthy Brain Book* by Drs. William Sears and Vincent Fortanasce.

Enjoy Music to Mellow Your Conquer-Cancer Mind

Yes, there is a scientific basis for the phrase "a sound mind." During Dr. Bill's healing from cancer he noticed that one of the most enjoyable "therapies" for getting his mind off his cancer and his discomforts was listening to music, especially melodies that triggered cheerful memories from the past. Was this just his imagination, he wondered, or was there science to support his feeling that music is good for the mind, especially during healing?

According to Dr. David Simon, former medical director of neurological services at Sharp Cabrillo Hospital in San Diego, California, you can measure the physiologic effects of healing music. Music, such as chants, triggers naturally occurring medicines called endogenous opiates that act as both pain killers and healing agents in the body. Music can lessen pain during healing, meaning less need for pain-relieving drugs.

Music meditation also clears the mind of toxic thoughts, which psychologists have dubbed ANTs (*a*utomatic *n*egative *t*houghts), creating more cerebral real estate for healing feelings and thoughts.

There's more! Science shows that music also:

- Balances heart and breathing rates.
- Decreases anxiety, and mellows moods.
- Lowers blood pressure.
- Increases interleukin-1, an immune-system regulator.
- Lowers the stress hormone cortisol.
- Fosters more quality sleep in pre-op patients.

Dr. Bill notes: *During my hospital healing from colon-cancer surgery, Martha played Strauss waltzes, and in my mind I replayed scenes of us ballroom dancing. I've also seen the healing power of music in the operating room. When I used to assist with surgeries, I noticed how much calmer everyone was when background music was played, from the surgeons to the unconscious patient (studies show that even during anesthesia, the auditory center of the brain still picks up music).*

Be nice to your neuropeptides. Remember those "molecules of emotion," or brain chemicals that circulate throughout your body, carrying biochemical text messages? The cells of the lining of your intestines, which are rich with receptors for these chemicals (this may be the basis of the term "gut feelings"!), are easily influenced by sound waves in music—just another way music helps balance the anti-cancer mind.

<hr>

Pick Your Music Before Surgery

Continuing with our theme of "music helps you feel well to heal well," we recommend selecting your favorite calming music before going to the hospital for surgery. Then play your songs in your hospital room right up to surgery and during recovery. Our personal pick: music medleys by pop and classical pianist Emile Pandolfi.

<hr>

Enjoy Nature Therapy

See Chapter 6 on how movement, nature, and especially movement in nature is medicine for the conquer-cancer mind.

Deep Breathe Cancer Away

We all know Dr. Mom's wise direction to "take a deep breath" to quiet the mind when we're overstressed, yet digging deeper into the research we found that, at least theoretically, it could also calm the stress of cancer.

Not breathing deeply enough means the lower parts of your lungs don't open and, theoretically, the oxygen level in your blood falls. When your brain senses it's not getting enough oxygen, it gets stressed out. It messages your adrenal glands, which react by pumping out stress hormones to increase your heart rate and blood pressure, to get more oxygenated blood to the body.

When you stop and take a few slow and gentle deep breaths instead, it expands your lungs to better oxygenate your blood. Your heart rate and blood pressure lower. The level of stress hormones in your body returns to normal.

What really sold us on the value of periodic deep breathing was that cancer cells thrive in an oxygen-starved environment, so that's the last thing we want our bodies to have.

Dr. Bill notes: *I have a close friend who is a shallow, fast breather and also seems to be "on edge" most of the time. This correlation made sense. Her stress hormones are always revved up because her oxygen levels are down.*

Grow Your God Center—Help Heal Your Cancer

"People want to *feel good* and *feel God*" is one of our favorite quotes from one of our most trusted brain scientists, Dr. Candace Pert.

Oncologists have noticed, and scientific studies confirm, that the deeper a person's spiritual belief, the greater their healing—what we call *the God effect*. You already know that building your conquer-cancer mind means devoting more cerebral real estate (aka brainspace) to healing. Another valuable healing tool is to grow your Godspace.

The science of "neurotheology" has found that the more frequently and deeply a person devotes their attention, prayer, and meditation to their belief in a personal higher power, the bigger the centers of the brain devoted to hope, wellness, and conquering cancer (that is, their God center) grow. While neuroscientists don't yet know how this happens, we believe that the Godspace in your brain sends biochemical messages to your conquer-cancer army inside, prompting it to work smarter for you. This God effect also explains why "We're praying for you!" is one of the most welcome messages a friend can send to a person with cancer.

The usual replies when we ask someone with cancer how their spiritual practices help them heal are:

- "I don't feel helpless or hopeless!"
- "I can handle my cancer-worrying better!"
- "When I let God into my mind, I make better decisions."
- "I let go and let God!"

Spiritual growth deserves a place in your overall "fitness program" for conquering cancer, alongside mental and physical fitness. Reflecting on prayerful feelings such as "Dwell deeply in me, God," "Help me trust in you, Lord," and "Guide me, good God" helps close the window in your mind that lets in stressful thoughts, and opens a window of tranquility, hope, and love.

It's very unlikely that stress "caused" your cancer, but prolonged, unresolved stress can definitely sabotage your healing. Don't let it! A crash course in mind management will not only help you heal from cancer but also carry over into your "new normal" for living a healthier and happier life.

Stuff happens while you're coping with cancer. So many cancer contributors (such as toxins in food and air) are not fully under your control. Yet one top conquer-cancer tool is under your control: what thoughts you let take up space in your mind. This important fact is why we begin our book with how to have a conquer-cancer mind, and add a second helping on managing the mind in this chapter.

Chapter 8

Sleep Cancer Away

People with cancer who sleep better heal better.

While healing, the fear factor, the pain of cancer, and the adverse effects of some cancer treatments can sabotage a healthy night's sleep—just what you don't want. Why? While you are sleeping, your immune system army inside is working smarter to weaken the cancer cells lurking in your body and get rid of those renegade rascals. But that's not the only reason sleep is important. During quality sleep, your conquer-cancer toolbox opens.

Why Sleep Is So Healing

Quality Sleep	Poor Sleep
• Blunts high blood-sugar spikes	• Raises blood sugar
• Reduces excess belly fat	• Increases excess belly fat
• Balances stress hormone levels	• Increases stress hormone levels
• Makes more melatonin (see how melatonin fights cancer, page 151)	• Makes less melatonin
• Releases natural antidepressants	• Can lead to increased depression
• Can lessen the adverse effects of chemotherapy	• Can increase adverse effects of chemotherapy
• Strengthens your cancer-fighting army inside	• Weakens your cancer-fighting army
• Increases survival rate	• Decreases survival rate

One of the earliest red flags suggesting a link between poor sleep and more cancer was the observation that night shift workers had a much higher incidence of many cancers, especially breast cancer. Delving into the "why" behind this "what," researchers discovered sleep deprivation sabotages healing in two ways: it dampens the cancer-fighting ability of your NK cells, and it lessens the level of a top conquer-cancer medicine you make—melatonin.

Your immune system loves sleep. The deeper and longer you're asleep, the greater the quantity and quality of cancer-fighting NK cells you produce. Think of this as your immune system night shift arriving for house-cleaning. The more NK cells you have, and the stronger they are, the easier it is to heal from cancer.

During quality sleep, you dispense your own anti-cancer medicine. Melatonin, your brain's natural sleeping pill, is one of the most powerful antioxidants and anti-cancer medicines that your body can make. It triggers the off-switch in tumor genes, lessens blood supply to cancer tissue, and helps the cancer-fighting cells in your immune system army fight better for you. Studies have found that taking melatonin in combination with chemotherapy can help both improve cancer healing and lessen chemotherapy's adverse effects.

Sleep better, balance your body. Cancer happens when the body is out of balance, and one way the body gets out of balance is when it collects more carcinogens than it can dispose of. Quality sleep helps restore this balance.

Your body has a garbage-disposal system, especially in your brain, called the "glymphatic system." When you drift into a peaceful night's sleep, the brain's natural garbage collectors, glia cells, are ready for work in your brain. Like microscopic garbage trucks, they grab the waste products. Here's another "Wow!" The rivers of fluid flowing through your brain, called the lymphatic system (part of your immune system), widen during quality sleep. So, when you sleep, you have more garbage trucks available and wider rivers into which the garbage can be dumped.

Try These Tips to Sleep Better and Heal Better

Better Your Bedroom

As we learned more about how quality sleep is so cancer healing, we upgraded our bedroom to become our cancer-healing sleep sanctuary. You spend more cancer-healing time in your bedroom than any other room in your home. To help you get into a good night's sleep routine and design your own sleep sanctuary:

- Place your bed close to fresh air from open windows, weather permitting.
- Cool your bedroom to 60 to 70°F.
- Cool your thoughts each night before entering. Leave worrisome thoughts about the previous or next day out of your mind.
- Decorate the halls leading to your bedroom door with photos or art that make your brain say "Ahh . . . like!" and tape a few photos and love notes on the door. (Martha calls Dr. Bill's collection "lovies.")
- Remove cell phones, iPads, and computers from the bedroom at least one hour before bedtime, and dim your bedroom lighting at least a half hour before bedtime.

(See the related section on how to keep cancer contributors out of your bedroom, page 162.)

Dr. Bill's sleep story. *As I was healing from leukemia, I noticed that "I am tired" was a frequent refrain of mine throughout the day. Initially, I thought it could be an adverse effect of the chemo, since it's human nature to blame everything on the medicines you're taking. Yet, something inside me said that these prompts came from my inner wisdom. My body was saying, "Bill, you have leukemia—rest!"*

Around 9 o'clock, an hour earlier than my usual before-cancer bedtime, I would feel a biochemical nag, as if my body were giving me marching orders to go to sleep. When I listened to it and went to sleep when my wise body told me to, I slept better. When I dumbly didn't listen in order to finish what I was doing, or check my email one more time, or stay longer at a party, I didn't sleep as well that night.

In studying what I had experienced, I found that there is a term for this internal prompt. Neuroscientists call it "sleep pressure." Listen to it as much as you can!

Three years later, I still enjoy the cancer-prompt that helped train me: "Earlier to bed and earlier to rise triggers cancer's demise."

Pay Attention to Your Inner Sleep Prompts

Journal your personal "nag time," that inner prompt that tells you "Time for bed!" As often as possible, aim to hit the sack when that inner nag nudges. For example, if your sleep prompt usually occurs between 9:30 and 10:00 PM, plan to start winding down for bed at 9:00 PM.

Consult a Sleep Specialist

The quality sleep–conquer-cancer connection is a good reason to add a sleep specialist to your team of cancer-care providers.

More Sleep-Well Tips

For our best advice on how to get a healthier night's sleep, see *The Healthy Brain Book* and our thirty-page program at AskDrSears .com/sleep-well-tips.

Get Less Cancer or More Cancer—It's Your Choice!

In surveying the scientific studies on who gets more or less cancer, the following "nice list" and "naughty list" items pop up most often:

"Nice List"	"Naughty List"
• Eats more plant-based and less animal-based foods	• Eats more animal-based foods and less plant-based foods
• Exercises habitually	• Sits too much
• Has a lean waist and low body fat	• Is overweight or obese
• Meditates more, agitates less	• Worries too much
• Doesn't smoke	• Smokes
• Drinks less alcohol	• Drinks excess alcohol

Chapter 9

Live Cleaner, Get Less Cancer

Many of us live in an environment full of toxins—*grow-food for cancer.*

Many cancers are caused by exposing the body to more "garbage," such as environmental toxins or carcinogens, than its garbage-disposal system (the immune system) can handle. Bad guys overwhelm the good guys and you get cancer!

The solution? Live clean! Besides strengthening your immune system, to get less cancer, minimize your exposure to toxins.

Don't disrupt those hormones! In medical language, many environmental toxins are known as "endocrine disrupters." As you have learned, cancer occurs when your usually protective immune system experiences "hormonal disharmony" or imbalance.

L.E.A.N. out pesticides. One of the most prevalent carcinogens, pesticides (also called persistent organic pollutants, or POPs) in the food we eat and air we breathe are also known to accumulate in body fat—another motivation to stay lean. And ladies, ponder this: Breasts are naturally fatty. Could this be why pesticides are such a big contributor to breast cancer?

Sprayed in America

Our passion for studying what we call "sprayed in America" began with Dr. Bill's leukemia and especially with Martha's breast cancer. We learned that many pesticides, which we come into contact with through the air we breathe and the food we eat, are considered carcinogens, and that the problem with pesticides starts with the gut.

To begin with, the pesticides sprayed to kill bugs on crops like wheat can also kill the good bugs in your gut. Don't spray your microbiome! (See more on the microbiome, page 17.) But that's not the only damage these pesticides can do. When pesticides and chemical fertilizers in food get into your gut, they can injure the tight junctions between gut cells. This injury causes your gut's protective lining to leak, letting those toxic chemicals into your bloodstream and the rest of your body, where they can cause your cells to turn cancerous. Pesticides can also damage the protective lining of the brain, the blood–brain barrier, and leak through into the brain. And some of these carcinogens have a "long half-life," toxin-speak for the ability to stay in your body for years.

Chemical pesticides and fertilizers also stimulate inflammation of the gut lining. Anti-inflammatory medications can treat this condition, but these medicines, if overused, are also gut-junction disrupters and can cause a leaky gut. This sick cycle continues: more leaking leads to more medicines leads to more leaking. *It's time to stop these leaks.*

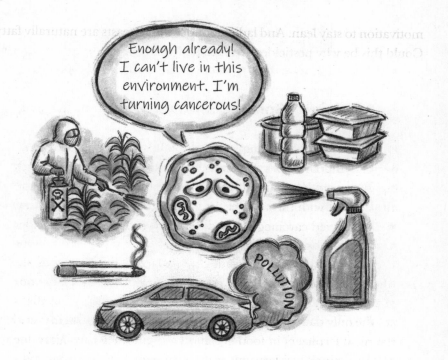

A Four-Part Plan for Cleaner Living

Of all our conquer-cancer tools, living pure is the most challenging to do, mainly because we live in a polluted world, where exposure to environmental toxins is not totally under our control. Yet, the following suggestions can help.

1. Know Your Naughty List

The first step to keeping carcinogens from getting into your body is knowing what toxins lurk in your everyday living.

The following chemicals, which can be found in our food and environment, are either known or suspected carcinogens. In some cases, our information about the health risks of these substances is incomplete, because internal studies funded by manufacturers are not made public.

- Aromatic amines (found in hair dyes, tobacco smoke, diesel exhaust, and textile factories)

- Arsenic (can be found in drinking water)
- Benzene (exhaust fumes)
- Bisphenol A, or BPA (found in plastic bottles and food containers)
- Ethylene oxide (found in household cleaners, cosmetics, and plastics)
- Fire retardants (used in some clothing)
- Formaldehyde (found in building materials)
- Nitrosamines (found in fried bacon and processed meats)
- Parabens (found in cosmetics, shaving lotions, and moisturizers)
- Perchloroethylene (used in dry cleaning)
- Perfluorinated compounds, or PFCs (used in textiles and food packaging)
- Pesticides and herbicides, especially glyphosate and atrazine
- Phthalates (found in solvents, vinyl, and plastics)
- Polyvinyl chloride, or PVC (found in plastics, cookware, and cans)
- Radon (a gas that can be present in poorly ventilated basements)
- Triclosan (found in toothpaste, dishwashing detergents, and soaps)

Instead of buying products containing these toxins, try to use substitutes. For more information about these substances and other chemicals used in our living environment, along with safer alternatives, see ewg.org and chemicalsafetyfacts.org.

Cancer: Made in America

Many carcinogenic products, especially pesticides, are banned throughout most of the world except—sadly—in the United States. Our government has bowed to the influence of Big Pesticide, and we are paying the cancer price.

Consider the cumulative cocktail effect. Even though a chemical may be labeled "safe" in animal tests, the thousands of pollutants we're exposed to in our daily diet and living add up. It is no wonder why our rise in cancer has paralleled a rise in our exposure to these pollutants.

2. Go Organic!

Consider these motivators to "go organic, get less cancer":

- **Children fed organic foods are less polluted.** A "wow!" study revealed that children who ate organic food enjoyed a lower level of pesticides in their urine compared to children who ate a conventional diet. Need more convincing? Another study revealed that children who previously ate a conventional diet and tested higher for pesticides in their urine tested pesticide-free after three days of eating organic-only foods.

- **Organic foods may be more nutritious.** According to a study done by the European Union called the QLIF (Quality Low Input Food) Project, organic fruits and vegetables contain up to 40 percent more antioxidants and higher levels of minerals like iron and zinc. Vitamin C is also higher in organic foods. (It makes sense that organically grown plant foods contain more antioxidants, since these plants experience more environmental stress and therefore need to make more of their own "medicines" to protect themselves from insects.)

- **Organic milk is healthier.** Milk from organic cows contains up to 90 percent more antioxidants and a healthier ratio of omega-3s to omega-6s.

- **Organic foods usually taste better.** Organic fruits and vegetables are approximately 21 percent higher in natural sugars, which may provide a naturally sweeter taste. One theory is that the chemicals in nonorganic fertilizers interfere with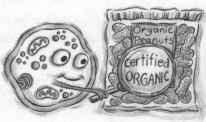

the plant's own metabolism. If fertilizers mess up the plant's metabolism, could they mess up ours?

Learn label loopholes. Products with the USDA label *"Made with organic"* may include as few as 70 percent organic ingredients. The label "Organic" means 95 percent or more. Also, look for the phrase "certified organic" and not just "organic," which ensures that no prohibited chemicals were used for three years prior to harvest. The labels "natural" and "pure" are meaningless and misleading.

The dirty dozen. Some plants accumulate more toxic pesticide residue than others. Download updated lists of the "Dirty Dozen" and the "Clean Fifteen" at ewg.org, and then tape them on your fridge or save them in your cellphone for reference when food shopping. These lists are from the nonprofit organization Environmental Working Group (ewg.org) and based on the results of nearly 50,000 tests.

What about genetically modified organisms (GMOs)? Answer: We don't know! Smart thinking: When in doubt, leave it out.

Dr. Bill notes: *Yes, going organic is more expensive, but so is cancer!*

Go Meat-Less!

Most cancer-thrivers eat less meat and enjoy a more plant-based diet. Studies reveal that the risk of breast and colon cancer is less in individuals who eat less meat. Our reasoning for joining the eat-less-meat crowd: Pesticides are stored in body fat. These animals are deliberately fed to increase their body fat. Therefore, we concluded: Not in our mouths! To enjoy a healthier meat treat, look for terms on the package like "100 percent grass-fed and grass finished" and "certified organic."

Grow Your Own Garden

While our family was healing from our cancers, we concluded that the vegetables we most needed and trusted could be grown in our own backyard. Besides our own dirt garden, we love our Tower Garden, developed by plant researchers at Disney World's EPCOT (kids like that!). Occupying a space only about three by three feet, it fits on balconies, patios, and even indoors, and you feed and fertilize it only with noncarcinogenic ingredients. We grab a handful of kale and parsley for our morning smoothies, and yummy lettuce, onions, and tomatoes for our evening salads. (See AskDrSears.com/TowerGarden.)

3. Do Your Daily Detox

The reality of modern living is that it's impossible to live totally clean. Yet, there are practical ways that most of us can lessen our exposure to environmental carcinogens. How clean you want to live depends on how much you value conquering cancer.

Start with the kitchen. In addition to eating organic, pesticide-free foods, do the following as much as possible:

- Drink from glass or ceramic containers instead of Styrofoam or plastic bottles.
- Buy foods stored in glass containers or frozen instead of in cans.
- Avoid plastic cutting boards. Use stainless steel or nontoxic wooden boards instead.
- Cook in stainless steel, ceramic, or cast iron pans instead of Teflon. If your so-called "nonstick" cookware is scratched from wear and tear, discard it.
- Heat in the microwave only in ceramic—never plastic.
- Replace plastic bowls, plates, and straws with glass, ceramic, or stainless steel.

- Store food in glass, stainless steel, or ceramic instead of plastic containers.
- Drink clean, filtered water (see ewg.org/waterfilters).
- Avoid cosmetics, nail polishes, and other personal-care products (sunscreens, shampoos, and toothpaste) that contain "parabens," a suspected endocrine disrupter, and other toxins (see safecosmetics.org).

You can also detox your home environment. Use the following guidelines to remove even more carcinogens:

YARD:
- Use only organic, environmentally safe sprays.

ENTRANCEWAY:
- Remove your shoes when you enter and change into home-based slippers. (You may have walked on pesticide-dosed grass!)

KITCHEN:
- Open windows for more ventilation while cooking with gas to lessen fume inhalation.
- Have your water tested for arsenic, lead, and heavy metals, and purchase a filter if needed.
- Stand a few feet away from the stove and use back burners, when possible, when gas is on.
- Stand at least six feet away from the microwave when it's in use.

BEDROOM:
- We spend at least one-third of our day in the bedroom, where we are "in touch" with and "in smell" of many possible carcinogens. See ewg.org for safer choices for your mattress, pillow, headboard (it can contain formaldehyde!), and more.

LAUNDRY:

- Be sure to ventilate your room to reduce inhaling toxic laundry detergent fumes, and see ewg.org for safer detergents.
- Hang recently dry-cleaned clothes (especially if covered in a plastic bag) to air them out for twenty-four hours before putting them in your closet.

AIR AND FLOORING:

- If you have a basement, have the air tested for radon levels.
- See ewg.org for suggested air filters and environmentally friendly plants to help purify your air.
- See ewg.org for environmentally safe floor, carpet, and surface cleaners.

Driving Cleaner

Breathe cleaner on the road, too! When possible, avoid getting behind or alongside diesel fuel exhaust–spewing vehicles. If it's impossible to totally avoid pulling in dirty air from outside, check the driver's manual in your car for how to recirculate cleaner air.

Initially, you may think, "Oh, this is too much work." Take more control of your environment by changing your thinking to "I'm living cleaner in an environment with fewer cancer contributors."

While we wouldn't want to live in a bubble and it's impossible nowadays to live in a totally clean environment, it's a good feeling to know that you can at least partially control your exposure to carcinogens. Remember, carcinogenic exposure adds up. Imagine you change your environment to lessen just twenty carcinogenic microexposures each day. Do the math: That's around 600 fewer microexposures a month, and 7,300 fewer a year. Many microexposures can add up to many contributors to cancer.

Learn More About Environmental Toxins

Because the overloaded world of environmental carcinogens is everchanging, for updates on carcinogens, brand names of safer products, and many other ways to enjoy a less carcinogenic environment, see the trusted resource Environmental Working Group at ewg.org.

Consult a Toxicologist

While you probably didn't think of adding a toxicologist or environmental health specialist to your list of other "-ologists," consider adding this specialist in carcinogenic toxins to your conquer-cancer team. They can become your partner in examining your habits and environment to identify possible contributors to your cancer and ways to lower those contributors' levels and exposure.

A toxicologist will:

- Go through your history of toxin exposures and identify the most carcinogenic ones.
- Define a cleaner living plan for you.
- Test your urine, blood, and other areas of your body for carcinogen levels.
- Prescribe a personal detox plan.
- Teach you what foods to buy and eat and how to prepare them to lessen your toxin exposures.
- Show you how to design a cleaner home using air filters, water filters, safer cookware, and more.
- Teach you what personal-care products contain the fewest carcinogens.

Even as a doctor and nurse we greatly undervalued how much exposure we had to cancer contributors in our environment until we consulted a specialist in this area to get help designing a detox plan.

Testimony from a Dietician Specializing in Toxin Testing and Detox

As an integrative and preventive practitioner with a life-long passion for finding the reasons for my patients' symptoms and diseases, I never thought I would be spending so much time testing patients for toxins and designing personal detox plans for them. The level of toxic metals, chemicals, contaminants, pesticides, and herbicides that have shown up and continue to escalate in my patients' testing results have shocked them and their families, as well as their practitioners and specialists.

One of my most recent patients, a woman in her fifties, consulted me for several health issues. Testing revealed high levels of toxins in her body and elevation of inflammatory markers. Additional testing revealed that she had early-stage breast cancer. As I went through her daily living and eating history, we found out that she was using lots of lotions, potions, and topical beauty agents. In addition, she mentioned she loved gardening and lawn care. She was using pesticides, including Roundup (the main ingredient is the suspected carcinogen glyphosate), and even spraying it on her bare hands without gloves to pull weeds.

Fortunately, after undergoing a lumpectomy for her breast cancer and following our detox plan, she is now leading a healthier and more vibrant life.

—Valerie A. Sayre, RD, LDN, RPhT
nutritionconnectionbalance.com

4. Sweat It Out!

Sweating is one of your body's natural waste removal systems for toxins. When possible, work up a sweat when exercising. Another great way to work up a sweat: enjoy the relaxing and detoxing effects of a sauna or steam room.

Science-based anti-cancer effects of heat therapy include:

- A healthier immune system.
- Better blood-sugar balance.
- Increased antioxidant activity.
- Better blood flow.
- Decreased storage of carcinogens in fat tissue.

Heating up and sweating in a ten-minute steam room session an average of four times a week got high priority in Dr. Bill's conquer-cancer plan.

Steam Your NK Team

Norwegian folklore has long praised the healing effects of saunas, hot baths, and steam rooms. Science agrees. Increasing your body temperature has been shown to increase your number of NK cells. People with cancer, especially those with compromised immune systems from chemotherapy, who enjoy more heat therapy usually heal better. Think: Heat can be healing.

While the science is soft, heat therapy may be healing because it mimics the effects of exercise on the immune system. As your body temperature increases, so does your heart rate and blood flow, which, as you learned on pages 126–127, mobilizes white blood cells, moving them from your blood vessel walls into your immune system.

The relationship between heating up and feeling better may also be due to the relaxing effects of heat therapy. When you relax more and stress less, your immune system fights better for you.

Caution: Before enjoying any type of heat therapy, consult your healthcare provider, in case you have an underlying condition, such as cardiovascular disease, in which you would not want to heat-stress your body.

A World Without Cancer

We have a dream of a world without cancer. But to achieve that dream, we need a mindset change. While we all have cancer cells in our bodies and in some ways are all currently "living with cancer," we must not lose sight of the fact that we can also work to prevent the root causes of cancer, rather than just accepting cancer as unavoidable. Besides living cleaner yourself, make your voice heard with government officials and healthcare providers by advocating for cleaner living laws and social change.

Our three-part action plan for achieving our dream world:

1. **Fund the good guys.** Subsidize organic food growers (meat, dairy, and produce) and tax nonorganic foods. Enforce that "organic" means not sprayed with pesticides. Lobby government agencies such as the National Cancer Institute and heavily funded private cancer organizations to spend a much larger percentage of their money on prevention rather than treatment. Devote resources to removing cancer-contributing pollution from our environment.

2. **Defund the bad guys.** We could "round up" a million concerned citizens to march on Washington shouting: "Prohibit cancer-causing chemicals!" The government learns a lesson. America becomes cleaner—and gets less cancer. Lobby to shift food-policy decisions from the Department of Agriculture (whose role is strictly economic development and not health) to the National Institutes of Health (NIH).

3. **Start clean-eating education in schools.** The most vulnerable—our children—are the ones who are getting the least education. Start teaching students beginning around the second or third grade about their immune system army and how to make it smarter—in a way that rivets their attention and motivates them to clean up their eating and living. At home, reinforce what children learn at school.

As a pediatrician for fifty years as of this writing, I plead to parents: grow your families in a less toxic environment. That is one of the greatest gifts you can give your children.

Your Daily Conquer-Cancer Guide

Even if you can't do—or stick to—all of the conquer-cancer tips in our book, do as many as you can for as long as you can. Remember the "cumulative effect" you learned on page 5—just as little doses of carcinogens accumulate over time and eventually "cause cancer," little changes can add up to a lot of cancer healing.

See AskDrSears.com/conquer-cancerguide for a one-page, full-color list of reminders (or see the black-and-white version on page 170), and how to rate your progress. Hang this guide throughout your home and office, and make it your cellphone wallpaper. Glance at it daily as a reminder and motivator to stay on your personal path to healing.

Then, at least once a week, rate yourself from 1 to 5 (5 being your best effort to follow our conquer-cancer suggestions) using the included list. Be honest! Visualize your progress—how well are you moving up from a 1 to a 4 or 5?

Action Items	How Well Are You Doing?
Believe you will heal (page 11).	
Smarten your ISA (page 29).	
Wisely partner with your cancer-care providers (page 43).	
Listen to your "doctors within" (page 17).	
Eat a conquer-cancer diet (page 84).	
Take science-based supplements (pages 111–112).	
Is your omega-3 index above 8 percent? (page 112)	
Is your vitamin D level above 40 ng/ml? (page 113)	
Get and stay lean (page 121).	
Spend at least thirty minutes a day moving outdoors (pages 134–135).	
Manage your stress (page 139).	
Enjoy quality sleep (page 149).	
Live clean (page 155).	

Part IV

Top Tips to Conquer Colon, Breast, Brain, and Lung Cancers

As you have learned, these conquer-cancer tools will help you heal from any cancer:

- Believe you will heal.
- Smarten your immune system.
- Partner wisely with your cancer-care providers.
- Eat a conquer-cancer diet.
- Move more, sit less.
- Manage your mind.
- Sleep cancer away.
- Live cleaner.

Yet there are additional tools that will help you deal with four of the most common cancers: colon, breast, brain, and lung.

Chapter 10

Help Heal Yourself from Colon Cancer

C olon cancer, especially colorectal cancer, is one of the most preventable, early detectable, and treatable cancers, and it gets our top vote as the cancer most "healable" using our plan. Consider the following top colon-cancer contributors:

- Carcinogens in food
- Excess wear and tear on the intestinal lining
- Years of eating foods that weaken the immune system
- Hard, sluggish bowel movements that press on the intestinal lining
- Unmanaged stress that weakens the intestinal tissue and protective microbiome living there

Our conquer-cancer plan helps reduce all these colon-cancer contributors.

Lifestyle is more cancer-contributing than genetics. Three members of the Sears family had colon cancer. A family history of colon cancer like ours should prompt genetic counseling and testing to determine if any of the cancer risk is inherited, and therefore suggest earlier and more frequent screening (see page 180). However, genetics plays a role in only 10 percent of colon cancer. That means 90 percent of colon cancer is caused by environmental factors, and might be prevented with the help of our L.E.A.N. conquer-cancer tools.

An observation that emphasized the importance of diet and lifestyle was the discovery that Chinese and Japanese people have a much lower incidence of colorectal cancer than Americans. Yet, when they move to America—and begin eating and living like Americans—they get colorectal cancer at nearly the same rate Americans do.

Dr. Bill's Good-Gut Health Program: Eat Cleaner, More Gut-Friendly Foods

When I was first diagnosed with colorectal cancer and designing my personal cancer healing program, along with reading up on what science said about colon cancer, I started with common sense. Colon-lining cells are known as "rapid turnover cells," meaning they are replaced by fresh cells every week or so. That sounds like good news. Yet the faster cells grow, the more prone they are to turning cancerous. Therefore, "protect those precious colon-lining cells" became my focus, as part of my larger goal of making colon health my hobby. I'm just sorry it took colon cancer to convince me to do so!

As much as possible I tried to eat foods that were the least polluted with environmental carcinogens:

- I decided no pesticide-poisoned foods would wind up in my gut. I went organic according to the "Clean Fifteen" and "Dirty Dozen" you learned about on page 160. I became an online fan of the Environmental Working

---

Group and would frequently check what they had to say about the safety of a food before I would eat it.

- I began carefully reading labels. All those chemical ingredients, such as those ending in "-ate," were on my naughty list. If I couldn't find information about the preservative, flavor enhancer, and so on, I wouldn't eat it. In my reading, I discovered that most of the chemicals added to our foods *were never tested for safety*—a carcinogenic flaw in our system. Therefore, I practiced:

When in doubt, leave it out!

I also emphasized gut-friendly foods, which led me to eat, simply put, a *real-food diet*. As much as possible, I ate foods that went directly from organic farms to my table without passing through a processing plant. I became mostly a *pesco-vegetarian*. That means I ate:

- 80 percent plant-based foods.
- 10 to 15 percent safe seafood (see examples, page 89).
- 5 to 10 percent other animal-based foods, such as organic eggs, unsweetened organic whole-milk kefir and yogurt, and an occasional treat of wild game, like venison. (See an example of my daily diet, pages 117–118.)
- At least 40 grams of fiber daily.

I've been eating this way since 1997 and, as a result, I continue to enjoy good health and vibrant energy, even as I am currently healing from chronic myeloid leukemia.

The Better You Poo, the Less Colon Cancer for You

Besides cleaning up the foods that came into contact with his colon lining, Dr. Bill next took a self-constructed course in "poopology." It's not only *what* and *how* Americans eat but also what happens next that contributes to colon cancer.

Dr. Bill notes: *You would think that something that our colons do every day—poo— would be something a doctor would know more about. But, I didn't—until colon cancer caused me to become a "Dr. Poo."*

The softer, smaller, and faster our "leftovers" pass through our colon, the less pressure and cancer-contributing wear and tear to the colon lining. Americans tend to be constipated. Constipation and colon cancer both start with "C." Any correlation? We think so!

Ideally, you want the food to come in and get quickly digested, the nutrients to be absorbed, the colon microbiome to have its fiber feast, and then the remains to be evacuated in a timely manner, before they have a chance to irritate the colon tissue. The less time food residue stays in your colon, the better you heal from colorectal cancer and the less likely the cancer will recur. In and out keeps cancer out!

Here are a few ways to make your stools more colon-friendly:

The better you chew, the better you poo. Americans are a society of gorgers and we are paying the carcinogenic price. "Chew-chew times two" (as you learned in Chapter 5) and "the better you chew, the better you poo" are phrases I use to make colon-health points in my medical practice. Kids laugh; parents blush and smile.

The more mastication you do in the top end (your mouth), the less wear and tear (that is, colon cancer) in the bottom end (your colon). Many of the conquer-cancer foods listed on page 84 require a lot of chewing. That's a good thing! Chewy foods have lots of fiber, and fiber is colon-friendly. Fiber-rich foods, especially the raw vegetables in salads, require thirty to forty chews.

Well-chewed food gets mixed with saliva, forming smooth, easy-to-swallow "goop." The longer you chew, the more "good goop" you make. Your intestinal tract likes that! When the goop goes down your esophagus into your stomach, your tummy registers "like!" as if saying, "My job is now easier." Also, taking smaller bites plus chewing more lessens gastroesophageal reflux (GER, or heartburn), a painful ailment that can affect people of all ages.

Taking more time to chew also gives your stomach more time to send its usual neurochemical message—called the gastrocolic reflex—down to your colon to say, in effect, "Prepare to evacuate what's in there now. More is on its way down."

Drink water more, poo more. For pleasant gut health, drink ½ to ¾ ounces of water per pound of your body weight a day. For example, if you weigh 100 pounds, you would drink at least 50 to 75 ounces daily. Your colon is your body's water regulator. If you don't drink enough, your colon lining sucks more of the water from your poo, resulting in hard poops—and more wear and tear on intestinal-lining cells.

Eat poo-friendly, high-fiber foods. The conquer-cancer foods listed on page 84 are also the most poo-friendly. They are high in fiber, and fiber forms the structure of your stool. The right balance of fiber and fluids helps make poo just the right consistency: soft, smooth, and easily poop-able. Fiber and fluid in food increase food's transit speed and decrease its time in contact with your intestinal lining. Think "fiber sweeps!"

According to colon-health researchers, the more grams of daily fiber you eat, the better colon health you enjoy. Makes sense! Fiber:

- Speeds chewed food through the intestinal tract.
- Decreases the time carcinogens remain in contact with the colon lining.
- Feeds your cancer-fighting gut microbiome, the community of bacteria that resides in your colon. (Recent studies suggest that having a healthy microbiome lowers the risk of colorectal

cancer; learn more about your microbiome by reading *Dr. Poo*, page 180.)

Smoothies "smooth" colon cancer recovery. Not only does a smoothie a day help keep colon cancer recurrence away, it also helps recovery from colon cancer surgery. This is how Dr. Bill learned this new way of eating! He wanted to have easy-to-pass, soft stools to baby his post-surgery colon. By blending all those fiber-rich fruits and veggies, he let the blender do the work of smoothing out his poop. Call it "stool-ade" if you wish. Read and do the sipping solution on pages 104–107.

Eat according to the "rule of twos." See how, page 98.

Improving Your Waste Affects Your Waist

Because with our poo-friendly eating plan you feel fuller faster, you are more comfortable eating less. And because you eat real, clean, fibrous foods, you also sugar-spike less. These lower your risk for all cancers by shrinking your belly fat. (See how belly fat can contribute to cancer, page 122.)

Move your body, move your bowels. Research shows that people who exercise for thirty to sixty minutes daily can decrease their risk of colon cancer by 30 to 40 percent. The more you move, the better the stool moves through your intestines.

Dr. Bill notes: *I notice the "sit more/stool less" connection while traveling on long plane trips. Sitting for five to seven hours or more, in addition to eating fewer colon-friendly foods and more colon-damaging foods, is a setup for a painful gut. The gut has a mind of its own, and it does not like sudden, drastic changes. When you violate the colon-health rules of eating, the gut shuts down, and constipation is the result.*

Don't Hold on to Stools!

If you feel like you've got to go, go as soon as you can. Holding on to stools—ignoring what your colon is telling you—can lead to constipation, more straining, and more wear and tear on colon tissue.

Go meat-less. Meat-eaters are more prone to colon cancer. Why? In addition to containing carcinogens due to pesticide-heavy farming practices, and having more carcinogens added from charbroiling (as you learned on page 100), meat has a slower intestinal-transit time than most plant-based foods. Remember, the longer a food stays in your gut, pressing on the gut lining, the more irritation it can cause. If you must "meat-in" instead of "meat-out" your diet:

- Eat only organic, 100 percent grass-fed meat.
- Marinate it (see tips for cooking meat, page 100).
- Cut it into smaller bites.
- Chew it longer.
- Partner it with salads and cruciferous vegetables.
- Limit it to twice a week or less.

Also, consider replacing land animals with seafood. Science agrees with our "fish over meat" recommendation. In one of the largest dietary studies ever conducted, the European Prospective Investigation into Cancer (EPIC) study, people who ate less meat and more fish were able to greatly lower their risk of colon cancer.

You may be wondering if there is such a thing as a perfect poo for lessening colon cancer. We believe so. It shares these features:

- *Soft.*
- *"Squeezy,"* meaning when your doughnut muscle squeezes the last of the poo out, it tapers into a "tail."

- *Frequent:* at least two or three times a day.
- *Brown:* not too dark, not too light.

We are a constipated society. We eat too much too fast, chew too little, sit too much, and strain too hard. Are you getting the (poo) picture?

Read—and Do—*Dr. Poo*

For more on the poo/colon-cancer connection and more healthy gut habits, read our fun and informative eighty-page booklet *Dr. Poo: The Scoop on Comfortable Poop.*

Get Screened Earlier, Get Cancer Treatment Earlier

The main reason colon cancer is so "curable" is because we have expert tools for early detection, especially screening for fecal blood and periodic colonoscopies. Precancerous polyps can sit there for years before turning cancerous, which is why early detection and early removal can be lifesaving. While fecal blood testing and a stool-based gene test (Cologuard) can detect some colon cancers, only colonoscopy—a painless procedure—can efficiently find and remove precancerous polyps. Routine colonoscopy is one of the greatest cancer-prevention tools in healthcare.

Oncologists estimate that timely screening for colon cancer could cut the death rate from colorectal cancer in half. That's the good news. The bad news is that colorectal cancer has been steadily increasing in *younger* people, most likely paralleling the increase in obesity at younger ages.

When to consult a gastroenterologist and begin periodic colonoscopies varies according to your age and risk. See cdc.gov/cancer/colorectal and gi.org/topics/colonoscopy for updates.

If you have a cancer-prone lifestyle and diet, we suggest you see a gastroenterologist as early as your thirties, especially if you are obese; frequently constipated; see blood streaks on toilet paper; have abdominal bloating; or experience unexplained fatigue, abdominal pain, and weight loss.

Chapter 11

Help Heal Yourself from Breast Cancer

reast cancer is the most thoroughly studied and heavily funded of all cancers. The good news is, thanks to modern surgical and oncology treatments, women are surviving and thriving longer, even though breast cancer is still occurring at an alarming rate. Around one in eight women get breast cancer in their lifetime, mostly during the postmenopausal years.

If only there were a magical medicine to lower the risk of breast cancer. There is! It's called *diet and exercise*. Cancer specialists predict that following the conquer-cancer plans in Chapters 5 and 6 could lower breast cancer by 50 percent in premenopausal women and 80 percent in postmenopausal women.

However, that risk doesn't lower to zero. When Martha was diagnosed with breast cancer, we both were stunned. She certainly did not fit the "profile" of a person who gets breast cancer. She had stayed lean all her life, breastfed a total of eighteen years (yes, you read that right!), eaten primarily our prevent-breast-cancer diet, avoided excess alcohol, and knew how to manage stress. She had none of the risk factors that science says contribute to breast cancer.

When Martha was given the diagnosis following biopsy of a suspicious lump, we collected the most credible science we could find to help her heal and prevent recurrence. While you've read all those conquer-cancer tips in Part I, here's a second helping specific to breast cancer, listed in order of what produces the greatest healing effects:

1. **Eat your veggies.** Science shows that women who eat a primarily plant-based diet enjoy the least breast cancer. And according to one of the largest women's health studies ever done, the Nurses' Health Study, the younger women start eating as Dr. Mom prescribed, the less their chances of getting breast cancer when they're older.

2. **Stay lean.** Staying lean is another of the most common preventers of breast cancer.

3. **Move more, sit less.** Studies reveal that women who exercise thirty to sixty minutes daily can reduce their risk of breast cancer by 20 to 30 percent. Especially in postmenopausal women, those who remain very active also heal better. Researchers attribute this "move more, survive longer" relationship to a more balanced immune system, less inflammation, and better blood-sugar levels. One additional possible mechanism by which movement aids preventing and healing: exercise can lessen the excess estrogen that fuels some breast cancers.

4. **Drink less alcohol.** See why, page 96.

5. **Smarten your immune system.** Research shows that women with breast cancer who had the smartest NK cell army inside survived the longest and healed the best.

Advice for Breast Cells: Avoid Blood-Sugar Spikes!

Breast cancer cells have many more insulin receptors—those tiny doors on the cell membrane that insulin opens to let in sugar—than healthy breast cells do. Our conclusion: Eat less added sugar, get less breast cancer.

How to Wisely Partner with Your Cancer-Care Providers for a Personalized Breast Cancer Treatment Plan

There are three stages of breast cancer treatment that require you to be a partner in making smart decisions:

1. Surgery. Lumpectomy is much simpler than mastectomy, but either way, the current science of breast cancer surgery is excellent. To do your part to improve your postoperative recovery, preload your immune system to decrease your chances of infection and improve healing (see how on pages 33–40).

We recommend asking for a *morning* surgery, if possible, for two reasons. First, your required pre-op fast is easier. Second, depending on the degree of surgery you are scheduled for, you may not need to spend an overnight in the hospital: just check in—pre-op/surgery/recovery—and then check out. Late afternoon surgeries are less time-accurate. They are more likely to result in an overnight stay in the hospital and consequently higher chances of infection.

Martha notes: *Thank God Bill is hospital-savvy. Originally, I was scheduled for a 3:30 PM surgery. Bill refused. We changed hospitals and surgeons and had a great experience. I had an 11:00 AM surgery, finished around 2:30 PM, was in the recovery room for a few hours, and then home by 7:00 PM. As I walked into* *my home-recovery nest, decorated with my favorite flowers, my delightful daughters cheered, "Welcome home, Mom!"*

2. Chemotherapy. Chemotherapy is usually recommended after your surgery heals. The science supports its use, but be sure to use our "questions to ask" suggestions on pages 57–58, and be especially careful in reviewing your doctor's answer to the "cohort" question on page 58. Ask your oncologist if there is good science supporting your chemo prescription, and if you're getting the chemo protocol that best fits you. (See Martha's chemo-saving story, page 60.)

3. Radiation therapy. Here's where you need to do your most homework and seek the best expert opinions, because this is where the science is somewhat shaky for some breast cancers. Besides some studies on radiation therapy being less scientific—such as "retrospective" chart reviews by number crunchers, the weakest type of scientific data—many are not personalized. Be sure to ask your radiation oncologist to discuss the latest studies on recommended radiation therapy for your type and stage of cancer, your age, and your general state of health. Before you get plugged into a protocol, we also recommend you seek second opinions from someone who specializes in breast cancer radiation therapy.

Dr. Bill and Martha's expert consultant story. After we partnered with our trusted radiation oncologist and formulated a plan that seemed to fit Martha, Dr. Bill found one of the top oncologist experts in America specializing in breast cancer radiation therapy. Before our consultation with this expert, we emailed him all of Martha's pertinent information and the exact number, strength, and duration of treatment sessions her oncologist wanted her to have. We then set up a phone consultation with this expert and our radiation oncologist to be sure they were on the same page. Our expert later called us and said, "Yes, I feel confident that your radiation oncologist answered all of my concerns and you're good to go."

Top Conquer-Breast Cancer Tips from a Top Cancer Specialist

A few months before Martha's cancer diagnosis, we held a family party at our home. Our daughter, Hayden, invited a guest, saying, "Dad, a friend of mine has a person you must meet, Dr. William Smith, one of the top breast radiologists in the world." After a walk around our yard, Dr. Smith and Dr. Bill had bonded. There was a depth of sincerity in this doctor, who shared he had dedicated the past forty-six years of his life to the specialty of breast cancer after, as an eight-year-old schoolboy, watching his closest friend's mother pass away from the disease. We didn't realize then how much we would soon need Dr. Smith's advice.

Later that evening, another guest said to Dr. Bill, "Bill, do you realize you were talking to one of the top breast cancer specialists in the world? He travels to university cancer centers all over America to consult on the most challenging breast cancer cases and train other oncologists on the latest science and techniques."

A few months later, when Martha got her breast cancer diagnosis, Dr. Smith became our top go-to guy for guidance on the most science-based path to her recovery. And when we began putting together this book, we asked Dr. Smith if he would review what we had written and add a few of his personal suggestions; he agreed.

Here are some of his top additional tips, learned over the course of his career, to help people with breast cancer survive and thrive:

1. Thoroughly record the results of your monthly breast self-examination. At some point between your twentieth and thirtieth birthday, you should consult a breast specialist on how to examine your breasts for suspicious lumps.

Do your breast self-exam at the same time each month, such as on day five to seven of your menstrual cycle, when your breasts are less swollen than before your period. Many women find it easier to do their breast self-exam in a shower with soap.

If you find a breast mass:

- Write down in a journal the date and approximate size of the mass you feel. Compare the mass felt to a known object, such as an aspirin, pea, or walnut.
- Determine the location of the mass. It helps to assign both a time-clock location (for example, at two o'clock) as well as its distance from the tip of the nipple.
- The vast majority of breast masses are benign. Many times, after a full menstrual cycle passes, breast glandular tissue or cysts grow smaller or disappear altogether.
- If there is bloody discharge from your nipple (sometimes seen as a bloody spot on your bra or t-shirt), immediately seek consultation from your healthcare provider, who will prescribe a mammogram.

During your self-breast exam, don't just feel for lumps. Also raise your hands over your head and look for any creases or breast "dimpling." If you see any that is new, seek immediate medical attention.

Remember, too, that it is extremely rare for breast cancer to present with pain. Just because the mass isn't uncomfortable doesn't mean it shouldn't be checked out.

2. Get the most accurate and informative mammogram. Get your mammogram at a cancer diagnosis facility that uses both 3D mammography and guided ultrasound. If possible, schedule your annual mammograms at the same breast-imaging facility. If you are still menstruating, it is important to schedule mammograms during the same time of the month every year.

Keep Your Own Mammogram File

While you may be promised that "the cloud" will store and offer immediate retrieval of prior mammograms for comparison, that may not always be the case. Previous mammograms are worth their weight in gold because they serve as a reference to identify new and significant breast changes. Especially if you find yourself moving to another state, gather your old mammograms on a disk or flash drive to present to your new radiologist at your new mammogram facility.

Avoid using any antiperspirant on the day of your mammogram or lymph node biopsy, especially those that contain aluminum trisilicate particles. If you've used an antiperspirant since your last shower, gently scrub your armpits and breasts before the mammogram begins, since these particles often cling to the skin. Also, avoid drinking caffeine for two weeks before your mammogram since, in some women, caffeine may affect the density of breast tissue and obscure reliable mammogram readings.

The mammogram technician will help position your body and breast to get the best imaging views. Try not to worry if you are asked to "return for more imaging," as this is common and usually does not result in worrisome findings.

3. When in doubt, ask for a biopsy. Most of the time, the mass you feel will be benign, typically just a cyst or breast fat—especially in younger women. If, however, the mammogram shows a mass that is not a confirmed cyst, insist on a biopsy, regardless of the mammographic findings. Mammograms are not always accurate, but they are currently the best initial screening tool we have.

Martha notes: *I was amazed at the new technology on my ultrasound-guided biopsy. I first saw how the ultrasound identified the mass and then watched how the ultrasound guided the needle (the size of a pencil) right into the mass for the biopsy.*

If your biopsy is positive for malignancy . . .

4. Avoid internet articles written more than three years prior to your diagnosis. The art and science of diagnosis and treatment of breast cancer has grown immensely over the past three years. Avoid reading older articles that contain needlessly pessimistic data, which will only increase your worry and sabotage your healing.

5. Take notes. Bring a scribe to your first appointment to make sure you don't miss anything, but bring your own notebook, too, because writing your own notes can be therapeutic.

Dr. Smith observes: *People I see for a first consultation who have already begun developing their own personal conquer-cancer plan (as Dr. Bill and Nurse Martha call it) get much more out of our initial visit because they come prepared with the right questions and know how to challenge me to give them the best answers. It's normal to be initially overflowing with resentment or shame. An organ they were once proud of has now "turned" on them. Those who come prepared seem to remain calm and focused, and their tears, when they come, more easily recede.*

6. Don't hesitate to seek multiple opinions. You may be surprised at the range of treatment options.

7. Be optimistic. Over my decades of partnering with patients with breast cancer, I've noticed that the ones who stay optimistic heal better. And I've learned that the most optimistic patients are the ones who:

- Have faith.
- Have a positive healing community.
- Practice gratitude for their life and those who are helping with their healing.

8. Volunteer. The "helper's high" that Dr. Bill and Martha talk about is truly a reality. A very good research study compared volunteer hospital "pink ladies" to an age-matched control group of non-volunteers. The three-year trial clearly showed that if a patient had ever volunteered in any clinical setting, their cancer survivorship over five years was about 60 percent better. Helping others heal helps you heal.

Testimonial: How a Husband and Wife Healed Together from Colon and Breast Cancers

I will never forget the look on the surgeon's face as he walked down the hallway toward me that day in November 2017. I knew something was wrong before he said anything. "Joel doesn't have diverticulitis as we originally thought." Tears welled up in my eyes as I waited for him to finish. "I'm sorry, Mrs. Herbst, but your husband has cancer."

With those few words, our family's entire world was turned upside down.

My husband was diagnosed with advanced colon cancer that had perforated the lining of his colon and entered his stomach. His diagnosis came as quite a shock to us. He was only fifty, and although his family had a history of heart disease that we monitored closely over the years, cancer was never on our radar.

Joel was determined to fight the cancer with every resource available to him. His motivation in his battle was our family. He trusted the Lord with his life, but he also wanted to do everything he could to watch our children grow up and to grow old with me. The initial steps Joel took in pursuit of healing involved two rounds of chemo and a round of radiation. Before beginning any treatment, we sought out multiple professional opinions from various cancer centers around the country. We were told by every doctor we consulted that without chemo and radiation, Joel had a very low chance of survival.

As Joel began his treatments, we continued to research complementary and alternative medicine (CAM) options as well. It was very difficult for me to wrap my head around the thought of Joel undergoing such harsh treatments, and I much preferred a more natural approach. Joel was open to CAM treatments, but he felt strongly that he needed to pursue every available option. At one point he told me, "Julie, we have to throw the entire kitchen sink at this! I will not be a good husband and dad if we don't do it all."

After a long year of grueling treatments, Joel's body was weary and worn, but we were beginning to feel some hope. His scans were looking good, although the tumor markers in his bloodwork continued to fluctuate over the next year. We watched those levels carefully, but we felt like we were getting a second chance at life together. That meant every bit of the fight had been worth it.

In 2019, life appeared to be back on its way to normal again when I was suddenly diagnosed with an aggressive form of breast cancer. I had received a clean report on my annual mammogram just ten months prior to my diagnosis. My first thoughts were of my children and my husband. Our kids had already been through so much; how was I going to tell them that I also had cancer? And Joel was still working to regain his own health. I didn't want to add any more of a burden to his shoulders, yet I knew we would approach my journey to healing the same way we approached Joel's: leaning on the Lord together.

As much as Joel's diagnosis had devastated me, my own diagnosis shook me to my core because I have dedicated my life to teaching health and nutrition. Healthy living was a huge part of my identity, and to receive a cancer diagnosis when I had worked to be so health-conscious was shattering to me. A self-proclaimed, recovering perfectionist, I combed through my life, searching for the source of my cancer. I felt that if I could weed it out, then I could protect my family from anything like this ever happening again. The Lord worked in my heart as I worked through this process. I found many areas where I could live more naturally and holistically, but ultimately God showed me that my life was so much more fulfilling when I released control and allowed Him to handle the details. I may never know the exact cause of my cancer (or Joel's), but we have chosen to live as healthily as possible and leave the rest in God's capable hands.

We are still on our journey to healing, but we have learned so much along the way. Although Joel's approach was more traditional and mine was more alternative, we have participated in many of the same treatments.

There is so much more to healing than the physical aspect. Battling something like cancer has a great emotional and spiritual component to it as well. Every member of our family was accustomed to a frantic pace of living—always working, always doing, always tackling the next project. The appearance of cancer in our lives brought our busy schedules to a screeching halt. We learned the beauty of slowing down to allow our bodies and spirits the time they needed to heal. We read countless books, and we kept our favorite music on repeat. We spent a great deal of time with our kids; our family grew closer than ever and faced both of our diagnoses as a single unit. Joel and I wanted to be strong for our children, but oftentimes we ended up receiving strength from them instead. We are so proud of our sweet kids.

We never expected cancer to be the story of our family. I don't imagine that anyone ever does. But it is our hope and prayer that our journeys will bring glory to God and give hope to others who are walking the same path.

—Julie Herbst, fitness instructor and wellness educator

Chapter 12

Help Heal Yourself from Brain Cancer

"Y ou've got brain cancer," you are told. You shift your mindset: "I'll make brain health my hobby," you think. That's what you will now learn to do.

Brain cancer is the most challenging cancer to treat because the thick skull that protects your most valuable organ also makes brain tissue more difficult for neurosurgeons to access. The good news is that modern guided imagery and brain-mapping can help guide your expert surgeon toward removing much of the cancerous tissue while leaving normal brain tissue intact. Targeted radiation oncology for brain cancer has also made big advances in achieving the same goal: killing the cancer cells while preserving the healthy tissue.

In partnership with your cancer-care providers, oncologists, and neurosurgeons, learn—and practice—our brain-healing plan:

1. Learn About Your Brain

Your "textbook" in making brain health your hobby will be
our partner book, *The Healthy Brain Book*. The more
you learn about your brain, the better you can take
care of it and help it heal. For example, once upon
a time it was thought and taught that we can't
grow new brain tissue. Not true! You can repair
and regrow brain tissue at any age. Our brain
health plan shows you how.

My brain-healing textbook.

The Healthy Brain Book

2. Tend to Your Brain—
the Greatest Garden Ever Grown

Think of your brain as a garden. The plants in your garden—your brain
cells—grow best when you water, feed, and fertilize them, and keep out the
weeds and pests. Top on your new brain-health plan is to feed and fertilize
your brain garden with smart foods and more healing blood flow, and to
keep out pests and weeds: neurotoxins and toxic thoughts.

3. Feed Your "Fathead"

Celebrate your new title of "fathead"! Your brain is 60 percent fat. That's
why you need smart fats to feed your healing brain (see page 210). Yet fat
oxidizes (turns rancid), so you also need to eat more antioxidants (see why
antioxidants are awesome, page 85).

4. Protect Your Blood-Brain Barrier

Your precious brain is protected by a one-cell layer designed to let in nutrients to feed your brain but keep out neurotoxins. Yet years of exposure to

neurotoxins and not-so-smart eating can lead to a "leaky" barrier that allows these toxins to pollute your brain garden.

5. Value Your Vitamin D

See page 114 for how vitamin D is a neuroprotectant.

Since your brain is the organ most affected, for better or worse, by what you eat and think, the sections in this book on eating smart conquer-cancer foods and mind management are top brain-cancer healers for you to learn and do.

Reread the section on smartening your immune system army (page 24) as well. Your brain is blessed with its own immune system army, which goes into high alert during quality sleep—another reason to put sleeping well high on your conquer–brain cancer to-do list (see page 150).

Kristin's story. *The Healthy Brain Book* was written on the job. While our precious daughter-in-law was healing from twenty-five hours of meticulous surgeries to remove most of her brain cancer, our whole family stepped up to help her learn and do her personal brain-healing plan. The science-based brain-healing plan in *The Healthy Brain Book* was our gift to her, and she is now five years post-surgery and healing well, without any recurrence.

Here's Kristin's story, in her own words:

I am currently surviving brain cancer. Nearly six years ago, I was diagnosed with an anaplastic astrocytoma, a grade 3 malignant brain tumor. Overnight, my world became a whirlwind, from doctor appointments, MRI scans, two brain surgeries, six weeks of radiation therapy, and thirteen rounds of monthly chemotherapy treatments, not to mention having to wean my eighteen-month-old son. Now, as I approach the five-year mark since my last treatment with no signs of recurrence, I'm excited to share a bit of my experience so far in the hopes that it may help someone out there with their own recovery.

The easy part was nutrition. I've always been a clean eater, so it wasn't hard for me to sort of ramp it up in the healthy-eating department to help boost my compromised immune system. At times, during the chemo treatments, I couldn't tolerate solid foods, so we had to get creative with healthy protein shakes, juices, and soups. I also made sure to stay consistent with good supplements like omega-3s, vitamin D, and a fruit and vegetable concentrate; and I even kept a Crockpot of chaga mushroom tea going for extra antioxidants. It wasn't just for me; since I was extra vulnerable to catching illnesses from others, the whole family needed an extra healthy immune system during this time. Even my toddler ate his supplements (or "sprinkles") every day, to help lessen the chances of bringing home anything contagious from the park.

The hard part was my emotional/mental health. After getting over the shock of my diagnosis and what it would mean for me and my family, I struggled hard with stress, depression, and anxiety.

The biggest help was the wonderful support from my family. My loving husband went to nearly every doctor appointment with me, dutifully taking notes about everything, which freed me up to focus my energy on processing things emotionally instead of stressing about all the details of my care. My mom took care of our toddler during the weeks I spent in the hospital so that my husband could stay with me. My sister-in-law supported me by going to some appointments with me, sharing her own cancer experience, and just spending girl time with me. The times I couldn't get out of bed to do my mom thang, my husband understood and did his best to take care of whatever it was that needed doing. I would write down my recipes and he would make dinner while I watched shows or read to our son in bed. Those times of snuggling with my chubby little two-year-old were some of the best moments. We talked to him about my "booboo" and that he had to be super careful, and he understood as much as a toddler could. I think this has a lot to do with how he's grown to be so gentle and caring to others.

As curious as I was about my cancer, I heeded my doctor's advice and stayed away from doing my own internet searches about it. Instead, I asked as many questions as I could think of during my appointments, getting information straight from the expert on my case instead of scary statistics from

Google searches, which likely wouldn't have been accurate for my specific situation anyway and would have served only to fuel further anxiety.

Another big help was getting to know the hospital staff. I learned that radiation and MRI techs are some of the coolest people, and nurses can have the best senses of humor while having one of the hardest jobs in the world. I used to struggle with a severe phobia of needles, which made all the lab visits and MRIs incredibly stressful. But I found that getting to know the phlebotomists and other staff significantly helped.

I struggled a lot with some of the physical changes during my cancer treatments. But I leaned into them, turning them into something I controlled instead. After half my head had to be shaved for my first surgery, and knowing the rest of my hair would fall out from radiation and chemo anyway, I had my husband give me a buzz cut. Combining that with some winged eyeliner and lipstick, I totally rocked a look I'd been wanting to try but was unwilling to cut my elbow-length hair for.

My spiritual life was a huge part of keeping me going through this time. From daily Bible study and prayer to filling my room at the hospital with uplifting religious music, it all helped to keep me hopeful. Looking back, a lot of it seems like a messy blur, but I know God's hand was in everything.

One more important thing I did to help wrap my head around everything I went through was to create a box of mementos from my times in the hospital—things like an ID wristband, get-well cards, one of the glass bottles my chemo pills came in, a (deflated) balloon and stuffed heart that my husband gave me when we spent Valentine's Day in the hospital, and some prints from a photo shoot after my first surgery (I got dressed up all fancy with a flower crown to make my scar "pretty"). I put these mementos and photos into my "Cancer Box" and keep it stored in a closet. I look at it occasionally as one of my ways of processing what I went through and owning the experience. During those times when I'm feeling overwhelmed by it all, I can glance at the box and say, "Look at this. I did this! This was a real, extraordinarily hard thing, but I did it and came out the other side, and now I'm that much stronger." The box also helped in explaining the experience to my ever-curious son, who still thinks the MRI images of my brain are just the coolest thing ever.

Chapter 13

. . . .

Help Heal Yourself from Lung Cancer

E ven though the smoking/lung-cancer connection is now well known and tobacco usage has decreased, lung cancer remains in the top four of most diagnosed cancers, and it's no mystery why—we still inhale polluted air. The lining of your airways is vulnerable to exposure to carcinogens that you inhale with each breath. (Lung and colon cancers are so common for the same reason—both involve sensitive linings that are regularly exposed to carcinogens.)

While there are many dark sides to lung cancer, the one shining light is that you have so much extra lung tissue that surgical removal of your cancerous tissue still leaves you with enough lung tissue to enjoy normal breathing and living.

Use the conquer-cancer tools that you have learned throughout this book to achieve the top four goals of healing from lung-cancer surgery:

1. Overcoming post-surgery fatigue.
2. Growing new lung tissue.
3. Repairing damaged lung tissue.

4. Keeping the lining of your airways healthy, to serve as a barrier
    preventing carcinogens from leaking through and to help
    prevent lung cancer recurrence.

Eat better to breathe easier. Many people healing from lung surgery
will notice that now it takes more energy to breathe. To get enough air,
you may have to breathe faster and work harder, which uses more calories
and can leave the rest of your body feeling fatigued. The "medicine"? Eat
more of the nutrient-dense foods from Chapter 5 to help prevent the malnutrition and undernutrition that can accompany healing from cancer.

Movement makes healthier lung tissue. Movement is key to growing
new lung tissue and keeping your existing lung tissue healthy. Why?

1. The increased rate and depth of breathing that occurs during
    exercise strengthens chest muscles that have become weaker
    during the post-op rest period.
2. Movement increases blood flow to all parts of the body,
    including the lungs.
3. Exercise builds more tiny blood vessels (capillaries) in the lungs
    to help more blood reach, heal, and grow lung tissue.

Healing lungs like that!

Consult your oncologist and surgeon for what kind of exercises are
best for each of your lung-healing stages.

Help Your Aging Lung Tissue Stay Younger and Healthier

Older people are at greater risk of lung cancer occurrence and
recurrence because as we age so does the composition of our lung
tissue. The number of *air sacs* in the lungs (the tiny balloon-like
structures that fill up with air each time we breathe and transfer

oxygen to our red blood cells) decrease as you age. As the number of air sacs decreases, so does the number of capillaries surrounding them. This makes the transfer of oxygen from the lungs to the blood less efficient. Also, as we age, our diaphragm muscles become weaker, as do the small chest muscles between our ribs. Finally, our posture often changes as we get older, in ways that can cause us to take shallow breaths more often, instead of slower, deeper breaths. Both movement and deep-breathing exercises can help counteract lung-tissue loss as we age.

Breathe better to heal better. You probably have never paid much attention to "breathing better." Now you must! As you are healing from surgery, you may find that you naturally move your sore chest muscles less while expanding and moving your belly muscles more. That's good! You're already on your way to upgrading your breathing.

"Belly breathing" helps the lower parts of the lungs (which are larger and contain more air sacs and blood supply) inflate more easily. Use this better belly-breathing exercise until it becomes natural to you:

- Place your hand over your belly between your navel and ribcage. Feel your belly expand as you breathe in slowly and deeply through your nose (with your mouth closed) for a count of four. As you are nearing the count of four, gradually also expand your chest muscles within your comfort limits.
- Hold your breath for a count of four while your belly and chest muscles are expanded. This keeps the lower portions of your lungs expanded longer, to deliver more healing oxygen.
- Exhale slowly for a count of five or more either through your nose or through pursed lips. This slow exhalation also keeps the lungs expanded longer to deliver more oxygen.

After you master your new way of belly breathing, you'll notice that not only are you experiencing more energy and feeling more relaxed, but you are naturally breathing at a slower rate—say, between five and seven breaths per minute. The neurochemical connections between your brain and lungs are so finely tuned that you will eventually develop the rate and depth of breathing that is best for your healing.

As you get better at belly breathing, personalize the numbers of seconds you use to exhale. An initial count of four seconds is doable for most beginning belly breathers, but try to gradually extend it a few seconds longer—say, to the count of seven. As an added healing perk, having an exhalation phase that is longer than your inhalation one triggers the calming centers of the brain.

If that isn't enough motivation to continue this deep belly breathing, consider this: cancer cells thrive in an oxygen-starved environment. Supplying more oxygen to the microenvironment surrounding cancer cells helps prevent their growth.

Dr. Bill's Belly-Breathing Tip

To better enjoy the relaxing effects of slow, deep abdominal breathing, select your favorite two-word mantra to focus on as you breathe, such as: "feeeel" (inhale), "goooood" (exhale).

Move more and breathe better to heal faster. Bodily movements and deeper belly breathing trigger the lymphatic system—the system in your body responsible for detox—to increase lymphatic drainage from your lungs. This drainage helps remove more waste products of metabolism and also any pollutants from your lung (and other) tissue, clearing the way for more efficient healing.

Breathe Cleaner Air to Heal Better and Lessen Cancer Recurrence

Here's a refresher course on how to lessen the carcinogens that get into the air you breathe and also strengthen your airway's protective lining that helps kick out the carcinogens once they get in:

- Take inventory of what major and minor changes you need to make in your daily living to breathe cleaner air. Do you need to move to a cleaner environment, such as not downwind from a freeway or factories?
- Review driving in cleaner air, page 163.
- If you smoke, try to quit! Smokers have a twenty-five-fold greater risk of developing lung cancer compared with nonsmokers. The good news is that lung cancer risk drops substantially after quitting. There are many effective approaches to quitting, including nicotine replacement therapies. Talk to your health care professional. And if you are or were a heavy smoker (more than one pack per day for thirty or more years), you should get screened for lung cancer by an annual CT scan.
- Consider getting a consultation on air purifiers for your home and workplace. (See also ewg.org/healthyhomeguide /air-filters.)

Love your airway lining. Another way to help heal from and reduce recurrence of lung cancer is to keep the natural protective lining of your airways healthier. Let's take a trip down your trachea and into your bronchi to learn more about this magnificent protective barrier and how you can help it protect you from toxins.

The layer of your trachea and bronchi that is exposed to air is named the "mucociliary lining" because it contains two features: mucus and cilia. Cilia are like the carpet of the airway: trillions of little hairs growing from the lining that sweep back and forth. At the base of these cilia lie two layers of mucus. The mucus acts like an adhesive gel that traps germs and pollutants that get in your airway. Its buddy, the cilia, then fan upward to pump them up and out. This is called "mucociliary clearance." A healthy, protective airway has the right blend of mucus viscosity (trapping ability) and up-and-out movement from the cilia. When either of these mechanisms don't work at their best, more pollutants can get through into the cells of your lung tissue.

Two simple ways to keep your mucus and your cilia functioning properly are a "nose hose" and a "steam clean." Make your own "nose hose" saltwater nose drops (¼ to ½ teaspoon of salt to 8 ounces of warm water) or buy a pre-made saline solution at your local pharmacy or supermarket. Spritz a few drops of the solution into each nostril and gently blow your nose. Finish by "steam cleaning" your sinuses with a facial steamer for twenty minutes.

Dr. Bill notes: *In addition to its other health benefits (see page 110), garlic is a friend to healthy mucus production. As it is absorbed into the blood and excreted through the epithelial lining of the lungs, it stimulates the airway lining to secrete a watery fluid into the mucus lining, perhaps by a similar mechanism to the one that causes tearing, runny nose, and sneezing. Pulmonologists have long treasured garlic as a mucolytic, meaning it helps the viscosity of the mucus be just right for clearing the lungs. Some of our patients with deep coughs have found that breathing the aromatic garlic from hot, spicy homemade chicken soup loosens secretions and makes their lungs feel better.*

Keep well hydrated. Dehydration increases the viscosity of the mucus lining, which makes it harder for the cilia to sweep trapped pollutants out. Deep breathing in a steam room can help move the mucus along, at least in the upper airways; it would take very deep breathing to get that extra steam all the way down into the lower airways. Drinking enough water ensures your mucus stays fluid, which helps your cilia stay mobile. Remember, the more watery your mucus is, the less stuck mucus (and the pollutants it carries) accumulates in your lower airways.

Can Cancer Begin in Your Mouth?

Some dentists say yes. In his must-read book *The Mouth-Body Connection,* dentist Gerald P. Curatola cites the research showing that people who have more gum disease, or periodontitis, have an increased incidence of certain cancers, including pancreatic, kidney, head, and neck cancers and leukemia. That's why periodic visits to your friendly neighborhood dentist and dental hygienist to keep your gum tissues healthy are one more way to reduce your cancer risk.

Dr. Bill's daily oral hygiene regimen:

- Avoid antimicrobial mouthwashes.
- Avoid eating or chewing on sticky stuff, such as caramel.
- Swish periodically throughout the day with warm green tea.
- Keep your head straight instead of bent over ("text neck") as much as possible to promote good dental alignment.
- Always swish with warm water before brushing.
- Gently brush in the morning, after meals, and before bedtime with a warm-water softened brush.
- After brushing your teeth before bed, clean your tongue with a tongue scraper, clean the crevices between your teeth and gums with a proxy brush and dental floss, and water floss.

Cancer-Healing Recipes

The most motivated recipe designers are those fighting for their lives—or better said, eating for their lives.

During his cancer-healing journeys, once Dr. Bill had learned the most cancer-healing foods, he also had to discover enjoyable ways of eating them. His answer: Drink more smoothies and eat more salads, two ways of preparing foods so that they taste better and make it easier to sneak in foods he mentally didn't like but had to eat.

Below are the science-based smoothie and salad formulas Dr. Bill came up with during his personal beat-cancer crusade and continues to sip and eat most days.

Our Conquer-Cancer Smoothie Prescription

Select choices from each of the following five food categories. Start with a few ingredients that you already know you like, then gradually add more ingredients. Be sure to add *protein* and *healthy fats*, which will make your smoothie taste better and keep you full longer than a fruit-and-vegetable, carb-only drink. The percentage of nutrients in an ideal recipe is 20 to 25 percent proteins, 25 to 30 percent healthy fats, and 45 to 50 percent healthy carbs.

1. Healthy Liquids	2. Healthy Fats	3. Healthy Proteins
Kefir (organic, unsweetened) Coconut milk (unsweetened) Almond, cashew, or oat milk (unsweetened) Cow's milk (whole, organic) Goat's milk Green tea Organic juices: green vegetable, pomegranate	Avocado Nut butter MCT oil (organic) Coconut chunks Seeds: ground flaxseeds, hemp seeds, chia seeds, pumpkin seeds	Greek yogurt (organic, full fat, unsweetened) Nut butter Tofu Plant-based protein powder (for example, Juice Plus+ Complete)

4. Healthy Fruits and Vegetables*	5. Special Additions: Flavor and Additional Nutrients	
Berries: blueberries, strawberries Kiwi Papaya Banana Avocado Beets Greens: kale, spinach, chard, beet greens	Cinnamon Hawaiian spirulina Wheat germ Cacao powder Lemon or orange rind (organic) Ginger chunks (organic) Figs	
* For supermarket purchases, go organic whenever possible, especially for dairy products and the fruits listed on the EWG's "Dirty Dozen" list (see ewg.org/foodnews/dirty-dozen.php).		

Conquer-Cancer Salad

Choose from the four "food groups" below as you design your personal salad; I've listed some of our favorite examples of each. You don't have to pick from all four to begin with, but as you shape your tastes, you'll find you're able to add more. Eventually, as you learn what gives you good gut feel, you'll discover the ones that work for you.

1. Greens and Vegetables*	2. Seeds and Spices
Kale	Turmeric, with black pepper
Spinach	Pumpkin seeds (raw)
Arugula	Garlic
Red bell peppers	Rosemary, thyme, and oregano
Leeks	**3. Dressing**
Onions	Olive oil (extra virgin) and
Beet greens and root	balsamic vinegar
Broccoli	**4. Special Additions**
Brussels sprouts	4-ounce fillet of wild salmon
Red cabbage	Cheese: goat, feta, other favorites
Chard	Hard-boiled egg
Collard greens	Hummus
Asparagus	Beans, black or pinto**
Mushrooms	Lentils**
Tomato	
Edamame (raw soybeans)	

*For all salad ingredients, go farm fresh and organic as much as possible.

**If you suffer from *leaky gut syndrome*, your doctor may advise you to avoid legumes.

Dr. Bill's hot salad tip. *For a flavorful treat, prepare your salad, selecting your favorites from our recipe. Then, put the salad in a steam pan and steam for a couple minutes, or until the greens are wilted and the cheese is melted. Enjoy!*

Gratitudes

Huge hugs of thanks to our cancer-healing team! We are alive and thrive and are able to write this book because of your support.

Special thanks to Dr. Bill's oncologist, Dr. Richard Van Etten, Chief of Oncology at the University of California Irvine's Chao Family Comprehensive Cancer Center. Dr. Rick not only prescribed cutting-edge immunotherapy to heal Dr. Bill's leukemia, but also gave us bits of his wisdom throughout this book. Another hug of thanks to my internist Dr. Joe Nguyen for detecting Dr. Bill's leukemia during annual routine blood tests.

Our heartfelt appreciation to Martha's team of cancer healers: breast cancer surgeon Dr. Marla Anderson; oncologist Dr. George Miranda; and radiation oncologist Dr. Gene Fu-Liu. Our trusted team personalized her breast cancer treatment plan based on the latest cancer science and their expert caring.

To our extended family of prayer warriors and well-wishers, you all were there for us when we needed you.

Praise to our illustrator, Debbie Maze, who put her heart and artistic wisdom into making the text more riveting to read by pairing it with eye-catching and mind-remembering illustrations.

Thank you, Tracee Zeni, our diligent editorial assistant for more than thirty years. Additional thanks to our research assistants, Matthew Sears and Jonathan Sears, for their detective work finding the scientific articles that support our cancer-healing plan.

We deeply thank our literary agents, Denise Marcil and Anne Marie O'Farrell at the Denise Marcil Agency, for making the perfect match with BenBella Books.

A special thanks to the diligent staff at BenBella Books for their untiring patience and insightful suggestions: Leah Wilson, Editor-in-Chief, whose continued encouragement raised our writing to a higher level; Lydia Choi, Assistant Editor; Elizabeth Degenhard, copy editor; Jennifer Canzoneri, Marketing Director; Kim Broderick, Production Editor; Sarah Avinger, Art Director; Aaron Edmiston, Senior Production Design Associate; Adrienne Lang, Deputy Publisher; and Glenn Yeffeth, Publisher and CEO.

We thank you for your contributions to helping many readers thrive and heal from their cancer.

Recommended Reading and References

Chapters 1–4

Abbas, Abul K., et al. *Basic Immunology: Functions and Disorders of the Immune System*, 4th ed. Philadelphia: Elsevier, 2020.

Abrams, Donald I., and Andrew T. Weil. *Integrative Oncology*. New York: Oxford University Press, 2014.

Clark, William R. *In Defense of Self: How the Immune System Really Works*. New York: Oxford University Press, 2008.

Cuomo, Margaret I. *A World Without Cancer: The Making of a New Cure and the Real Promise of Prevention*. New York: Rodale, 2012.

DiNicolantonio, James, and Siim Land. *The Immunity Fix: Strengthen Your Immune System, Fight Off Infections, Reverse Chronic Disease and Live a Healthier Life*. Las Vegas, 2020.

Funk, Kristi. *Breasts: The Owner's Manual: Every Women's Guide to Reducing Cancer Risk, Making Treatment Choices, and Optimizing Outcomes*. Nashville: W Publishing, an Imprint of Thomas Nelson, 2018.

Kappel, M., et al. "Evidence that the Effect of Physical Exercise on NK Cell Activity Is Mediated by Epinephrine," *Journal of Applied Physiology* 70, no. 6 (1991): 25303–4.

Lichtenstein, P., et al. "Environmental and Heritable Factors in the Causation of Cancer—Analysis of Cohorts of Twins from Sweden, Denmark, and Finland," *New England Journal of Medicine* 343 (2000): 78–85.

Sears, William, and Erin Sears Basile. *The Dr. Sears T5 Wellness Plan: Transform Your Mind and Body, Five Changes in Five Weeks*. Dallas: BenBella Books, 2017.

Sears, William, and Vincent M. Fortanasce. *The Healthy Brain Book: An All-Ages Guide to a Calmer, Happier, Sharper You*. Dallas: BenBella Books, 2020.

Servan-Schreiber, David. *Anticancer: A New Way of Life*. New York: Penguin Books, 2009.

Chapter 5

Abdullah, T., et al. "Garlic Revisited: Therapeutic for the Major Diseases of Our Times?" *Journal of the National Medical Association* 80, no. 4 (1988): 439–45.

Aggarwal, Bharat, and Debora Yost. *Healing Spices: How to Use 50 Everyday and Exotic Spices to Boost Health and Beat Disease*. New York: Sterling, 2011.

Aune, Dagfinn, et al. "Dietary Fibre, Whole Grains, and Risk of Colorectal Cancer: Systematic Review and Dose-Response Meta-Analysis of Prospective Studies," *BMJ* 343 (2011): d6617.

Bayan, Leyla, et al. "Garlic: A Review of Potential Therapeutic Effects," *Avicenna Journal of Phytomedicine* 4, no. 1 (2014): 1–14.

Béliveau, Richard, and Denis Gingras. *Foods to Fight Cancer: What to Eat to Reduce Your Risk*. New York: DK Publishing, 2017.

Brasky, Theodore, et al. "Long-Chain ω-3 Fatty Acid Intake and Endometrial Cancer Risk in the Women's Health Initiative," *American Journal of Clinical Nutrition* 101, no. 4 (2015): 824–34.

Burton-Freeman, Britt, et al. "Strawberry Modulates LDL Oxidation and Postprandial Lipemia in Response to High-Fat Meal in Overweight Hyperlipidemic Men and Women," *Journal of the American College of Nutrition* 29, no. 1 (2010): 46–54.

Calder, Philip. "Fatty Acids and Inflammation: The Cutting Edge Between Food and Pharma," *European Journal of Pharmacology* 668, suppl. 1 (2011): 50S–58S.

Calle, Eugenia, et al. "Overweight, Obesity, and Mortality from Cancer in a Prospectively Studied Cohort of U.S. Adults," *New England Journal of Medicine* 348 (2003): 1625–38.

Calle, Eugenia, and Rudolf Kaaks. "Overweight, Obesity and Cancer: Epidemiological Evidence and Proposed Mechanisms," *Nature Reviews Cancer* 4 (2004): 579–91.

Davis, Brenda, and Penny M. Kris-Etherton. "Achieving Optimal Essential Fatty Acid Status in Vegetarians: Current Knowledge and Practical Implications," *American Journal of Clinical Nutrition* 78, suppl. 3 (2003): 640S–646S.

de Cabo, Rafael, and Mark Mattson. "The Effects of Intermittent Fasting on Health, Aging, and Disease," *New England Journal of Medicine* 381 (2019): 2541–51.

Duan, Wanxing, et al. "Hyperglycemia, a Neglected Factor During Cancer Progression," *BioMed Research International* 2014 (2014): 461917.

Etcheverry, Paz. "Vitamin D Can Reduce Breast Cancer Risk." *Life Extension Magazine*. July 2021. lifeextension.com/magazine/2021/10 /vitamin-d-breast-cancer.

Fernandez, Esteve, et al. "Fish Consumption and Cancer Risk," *American Journal of Clinical Nutrition* 70, no. 1 (1999): 85–90.

Galasso, Christian, et al. "On the Neuroprotective Role of Astaxanthin: New Perspectives?" *Marine Drugs* 16, no. 8 (2018): 247.

Garland, Cedric, et al. "Dietary Vitamin D and Calcium and Risk of Colorectal Cancer: A 19-Year Prospective Study in Men," *Lancet* 1, no. 8424 (1985): 307–9.

Garland, Cedric, and Frank Garland. "Do Sunlight and Vitamin D Reduce the Likelihood of Colon Cancer?" *International Journal of Epidemiology* 9, no. 3 (1980): 227–31.

Gerber, Mariette. "Fibre and Breast Cancer," *European Journal of Cancer Prevention* 7, suppl. 2 (1998): S63–S67.

Gerber, Mariette. "Omega-3 Fatty Acids and Cancers: A Systematic Update Review of Epidemiological Studies," *British Journal of Nutrition* 107, suppl. 2 (2012): S228–39.

Gray, Nathan. "High Levels of Carotenoids Backed for Breast Cancer Risk Reduction," nutraingredients.com, William Reed Business Media Ltd. 7 Dec. 2012. nutraingredients.com/Article/2012/12/07/high-levels-of-carotenoids-backed-for-breast-cancer-risk-reduction.

Grosso, Giuseppe, et al. "Nut Consumption on All-Cause, Cardiovascular, and Cancer Mortality Risk: A Systematic Review and Meta-Analysis of Epidemiologic Studies," *American Journal of Clinical Nutrition* 101, no. 4 (2015): 783–93.

Jafari, Mahtab. *The Truth About Dietary Supplements: An Evidence-Based Guide to a Safe Medicine Cabinet.* Las Vegas: Archangel Ink, 2021.

Khandekar, Melin, et al. "Molecular Mechanisms of Cancer Development in Obesity," *Nature Reviews Cancer* 11, no. 12 (2011): 886–95.

Khankari, Nikhil, et al. "Dietary Intake of Fish, Polyunsaturated Fatty Acids, and Survival After Breast Cancer: A Population-Based, Follow-Up Study on Long Island, New York," *Cancer* 121, no. 13 (2015): 2244–52.

Kim, Hyun-Sook, et al. "Dietary Supplementation of Probiotic Bacillus polyfermenticus, Bispan Strain, Modulates Natural Killer Cell and T Cell Subset Populations and Immunoglobulin G Levels in Human Subjects," *Journal of Medicinal Food* 9, no. 3 (2006): 321–27.

Kiremidjian-Schumacher, Lidia, et al. "Supplementation with Selenium and Human Immune Cell Functions. II. Effect on Cytotoxic Lymphocytes and Natural Killer Cells," *Biological Trace Element Research* 41, nos. 1–2 (1994): 115–27.

Knoops, Kim, et al. "Mediterranean Diet, Lifestyle Factors, and 10-Year Mortality in Elderly European Men and Women: The HALE Project," *JAMA* 292, no. 12 (2004): 1433–39.

Lappe, Joan, et al. "Vitamin D and Calcium Supplementation Reduces Cancer Risk: Results of a Randomized Trial," *American Journal of Clinical Nutrition* 85, no. 6 (2007): 1586–91.

LoConte, Noelle, et al. "Alcohol and Cancer: A Statement of the American Society of Clinical Oncology," *Journal of Clinical Oncology* 36, no. 1 (2018): 83–93.

Loomis, Dana, et al. "Carcinogenicity of Drinking Coffee, Mate, and Very Hot Beverages," *The Lancet Oncology* 17, no. 7 (2016): 877–78.

Mann, Denise. "Childhood Leukemia, Brain Cancer on the Rise." *MedicineNet*. 26 Jan. 2011. medicinenet.com/script/main/art.asp ?articlekey=125152.

McDonnell, Sharon, et al. "Serum 25-Hydroxyvitamin D Concentrations ≥40 ng/ml Are Associated with >65% Lower Cancer Risk: Pooled Analysis of Randomized Trial and Prospective Cohort Study," *PLoS One* 11, no. 4 (2016): e0152441.

Michaud, Dominique, et al. "A Prospective Study of Periodontal Disease and Pancreatic Cancer in US Male Health Professionals," *Journal of the National Cancer Institute* 99, no. 2 (2007): 171–75.

Michaud, Dominique, et al. "Periodontal Disease, Tooth Loss and Cancer Risk in a Prospective Study of Male Health Professionals," *The Lancet Oncology* 9, no. 6 (2008): 550–58.

Murff, Harvey, et al. "Dietary Intake of PUFAs and Colorectal Polyp Risk," *American Journal of Clinical Nutrition* 95, no. 3 (2012): 703–12.

Norat, Teresa, et al. "Meat, Fish, and Colorectal Cancer Risk: The European Prospective Investigation into Cancer and Nutrition," *Journal of the National Cancer Institute* 97, no. 12 (2005): 906–16.

Ornish, Dean, et al. "Intensive Lifestyle Changes May Affect the Progression of Prostate Cancer," *Journal of Urology* 174, no. 3 (2005): 1065–69; discussion 1069–70.

Ronti, Tiziana, et al. "The Endocrine Function of Adipose Tissue: An Update," *Clinical Endocrinology* 64, no. 4 (2006): 355–65.

Sánchez-Zamorano, Luisa Maria, et al. "Healthy Lifestyle on the Risk of Breast Cancer," *Cancer Epidemiology, Biomarkers & Prevention* 20, no. 5 (2011): 912–22.

Sears, William. *Natural Astaxanthin–Hawaii's Supernutrient*. 2015.

Sears, William, and James Sears. *The Omega-3 Effect*. New York: Little, Brown, 2012.

Seeram, Navindra, et al. "Blackberry, Black Raspberry, Blueberry, Cranberry, Red Raspberry, and Strawberry Extracts Inhibit Growth and Stimulate Apoptosis of Human Cancer Cells in Vitro," *Journal of Agricultural and Food Chemistry* 54, no. 25 (2006): 9329–39.

Sehgal, Amit, et al. "Combined Effects of Curcumin and Piperine in Ameliorating Benzo(a)pyrene Induced DNA Damage," *Food and Chemical Toxicology* 49, no. 11 (2011): 3002–6.

Song, Mingyang, and Edward Giovannucci. "Preventable Incidence and Mortality of Carcinoma Associated with Lifestyle Factors Among Whites in the United States," *JAMA Oncology* 2, no. 9 (2016): 1154–61.

Sun, Jie, et al. "Antioxidant and Antiproliferative Activities of Common Fruits," *Journal of Agricultural and Food Chemistry* 50, no. 25 (2002): 7449–54.

Szymanski, Konrad, et al. "Fish Consumption and Prostate Cancer Risk: A Review and Meta-Analysis," *American Journal of Clinical Nutrition* 92, no. 5 (2010): 1223–33.

Thakuri, Pradip Shahi, et al. "Phytochemicals Inhibit Migration of Triple Negative Breast Cancer Cells by Targeting Kinase Signaling," *BMC Cancer* 20, no. 1 (2020): 4.

Ugbogu, Eziuche Amadike, et al. "Role of Phytochemicals in Chemoprevention of Cancer: A Review," *International Journal of Pharmaceutical and Chemical Sciences* 2 (2013): 566–75.

Vanderbilt University Medical Center. "Eating Cruciferous Vegetables May Improve Breast Cancer Survival." *ScienceDaily*. 3 Apr. 2012. sciencedaily.com/releases/2012/04/120403153531.htm.

Vergnaud, Anne-Claire, et al. "Meat Consumption and Prospective Weight Change in Participants of the EPIC-PANACEA Study," *American Journal of Clinical Nutrition* 92, no. 2 (2010): 398–407.

Vogt, Rainbow, et al. "Cancer and Non-Cancer Health Effects from Food Contaminant Exposures for Children and Adults in California: A Risk Assessment," *Environmental Health* 11 (2012): 83.

Waladkhani, Ali Reza, and Michael Clemens. "Effect of Dietary Phytochemicals on Cancer Development (Review)," *International Journal of Molecular Medicine* 1, no. 4 (1998): 747–53.

Williams, Sarah. "Link Between Obesity and Cancer," *Proceedings of the National Academy of Sciences of the United States of America* 110, no. 22 (2013): 8753–54.

Zhang, Fang Fang, et al. "Dietary Isoflavone Intake and All-Cause Mortality in Breast Cancer Survivors: The Breast Cancer Family Registry," *Cancer* 123, no. 11 (2017): 2070–79.

Zhang, Shumin M., et al. "Alcohol Consumption and Breast Cancer Risk in the Women's Health Study," *American Journal of Epidemiology* 165, no. 6 (2007): 667–76.

Zheng, Ju-Sheng, et al. "Intake of Fish and Marine n-3 Polyunsaturated Fatty Acids and Risk of Breast Cancer: Meta-Analysis of Data from 21 Independent Prospective Cohort Studies," *BMJ* 346 (2013): f3706.

Zhu, Guoqing, et al. "Effects of Exercise Intervention in Breast Cancer Survivors: A Meta-Analysis of 33 Randomized Controlled Trials," *OncoTargets and Therapy* 9 (2016): 2153–68.

Chapter 6

Ashcraft, Kathleen, et al. "Efficacy and Mechanisms of Aerobic Exercise on Cancer Initiation, Progression, and Metastasis: A Critical Systematic Review of *In Vivo* Preclinical Data," *Cancer Research* 76, no. 14 (2016): 4032–50.

Ballard-Barbash, Rachel, et al. "Physical Activity, Biomarkers, and Disease Outcomes in Cancer Survivors: A Systematic Review," *Journal of the National Cancer Institute* 104, no. 11 (2012): 815–40.

Chlebowski, Rowan, et al. "Dietary Fat Reduction and Breast Cancer Outcome: Interim Efficacy Results from the Women's Intervention Nutrition Study," *Journal of the National Cancer Institute* 98, no. 24 (2006): 1767–76.

Connealy, Leigh E. *The Cancer Revolution: A Groundbreaking Program to Reverse and Prevent Cancer*. Boston: Da Capo Press, 2017.

Cross, M. C., et al. "Endurance Exercise with and Without a Thermal Clamp: Effects on Leukocytes and Leukocyte Subsets," *Journal of Applied Physiology (1985)* 81, no. 2 (1996): 822–9.

Ely, Brett, et al. "Aerobic Performance Is Degraded, Despite Modest Hyperthermia, in Hot Environments," *Medicine and Science in Sports and Exercise* 42, no. 1 (2010): 135–41.

Febbraio, Mark. "Alterations in Energy Metabolism During Exercise and Heat Stress," *Sports Medicine* 31, no. 1 (2001): 47–59.

Friedenreich, Christine, and Marla Orenstein. "Physical Activity and Cancer Prevention: Etiologic Evidence and Biological Mechanisms," *Journal of Nutrition* 132, suppl. 11 (2002): 3456S–64S.

Fung, Jason. *The Cancer Code: A Revolutionary New Understanding of a Medical Mystery*. New York: HarperCollins, 2020.

Galloway, Stuart, and Ronald Maughan. "Effects of Ambient Temperature on the Capacity to Perform Prolonged Cycle Exercise in Man," *Medicine and Science in Sports and Exercise* 29, no. 9 (1997): 1240–9.

George, Stephanie, et al. "Postdiagnosis Diet Quality, the Combination of Diet Quality and Recreational Physical Activity, and Prognosis After Early-Stage Breast Cancer," *Cancer Causes Control* 22, no. 4 (2011): 589–98.

Gleeson, Michael, et al. *Exercise Immunology*. New York: Routledge, 2013.

González-Alonso, José, et al. "Influence of Body Temperature on the Development of Fatigue During Prolonged Exercise in the Heat," *Journal of Applied Physiology (1985)* 86, no. 3 (1999): 1032–39.

Holmes, Michelle, et al. "Physical Activity and Survival After Breast Cancer Diagnosis," *JAMA* 293, no. 20 (2005): 2479–86.

Johannsen, Neil, et al. "Association of White Blood Cell Subfraction Concentration with Fitness and Fatness," *British Journal of Sports Medicine* 44, no. 8 (2010): 588–93.

Krüger, Karsten, et al. "Exercise Affects Tissue Lymphocyte Apoptosis via Redox-Sensitive and Fas-Dependent Signaling Pathways," *AJP Regulatory Integrative and Comparative Physiology* 296, no.5 (2009): R1518–27.

Lee, I-Min. "Physical Activity and Cancer Prevention—Data from Epidemiologic Studies," *Medicine and Science in Sports Exercise* 35, no. 11 (2003): 1823–27.

Maddock, Richard, et al. "Vigorous Exercise Increases Brain Lactate and Glx (Glutamate+Glutamine): A Dynamic 1H-MRS Study," *Neuroimage* 57, no. 4 (2011): 1324–30.

Mars, Maurice, et al. "High Intensity Exercise: A Cause of Lymphocyte Apoptosis?" *Biochemical Biophysical Research Communications* 249, no. 2 (1998): 366–70.

Maruti, Sonia, et al. "A Prospective Study of Age-Specific Physical Activity and Premenopausal Breast Cancer," *Journal of the National Cancer Institute* 100, no. 10 (2008): 728–37.

McFarlin, Brian, et al. "Chronic Resistance Exercise Training Improves Natural Killer Cell Activity in Older Women," *The Journals of Gerontology: Series A* 60, no.10 (2005): 1315–18.

Meyerhardt, Jeffrey, et al. "Physical Activity and Survival After Colorectal Cancer Diagnosis," *Journal of Clinical Oncology* 24, no. 22 (2006): 3527–34.

Nicholson, John, and David Case. "Carboxyhemoglobin Levels in New York City Runners," *The Physician and Sportsmedicine* 11, no. 3 (1983): 134–38.

Nieman, David, et al. "Effects of High- vs. Moderate-Intensity Exercise on Natural Killer Cell Activity," *Medicine and Science in Sports and Exercise* 25, no. 10 (1993): 1126–34.

Ortega, Eduardo, et al. "Stimulation of the Phagocytic Function of Neutrophils in Sedentary Men After Acute Moderate Exercise," *European Journal of Applied Physiology and Occupational Physiology* 66, no. 1 (1993): 60–64.

Pedersen, Bente, et al. "Natural Killer Cell Activity in Peripheral Blood of Highly Trained and Untrained Persons," *International Journal of Sports Medicine* 10, no. 2 (1989): 129–31.

Pedersen, Bente, and Henrik Ullum. "NK Cell Response to Physical Activity: Possible Mechanisms of Action," *Medicine and Science in Sports and Exercise* 26, no. 2 (1994): 140–46.

Pedersen, Line, et al. "Voluntary Running Suppresses Tumor Growth Through Epinephrine- and IL-6-Dependent NK Cell Mobilization and Redistribution," *Cell Metabolism* 23, no. 3 (2016): 554–62.

Simpson, Richard, et al. "High-Intensity Exercise Elicits the Mobilization of Senescent T Lymphocytes into the Peripheral Blood Compartment in Human Subjects," *Journal of Applied Physiology (1985)* 103, no. 1 (2007): 396–401.

"This is Your Brain on Exercise." *UC Davis Health Newsletter.* 17 Mar. 2016. universityofcalifornia.edu/news/your-brain-exercise.

Van Eeden, Stephan, et al. "Expression of the Cell Adhesion Molecules on Leukocytes That Demarginate During Acute Maximal Exercise," *Journal of Applied Physiology (1985)* 86, no. 3 (1999): 9707–6.

Walsh, Neil, et al. "Position Statement. Part One: Immune Function and Exercise," *Exercise Immunology Review* 17 (2011): 6–63.

Woods, Jeffrey, et al. "Effects of Maximal Exercise on Natural Killer (NK) Cell Cytotoxicity and Responsiveness to Interferon-Alpha in the Young and Old," *The Journals of Gerontology: Series A* 53, no. 6 (1998): B430–37.

Chapter 7

Anderson, Barbara, et al. "Psychological, Behavioral, and Immune Changes After a Psychological Intervention: A Clinical Trial," *Journal of Clinical Oncology* 22, no. 17 (2004): 3570–80.

Antoni, Michael, et al. "The Influence of Bio-Behavioural Factors on Tumour Biology: Pathways and Mechanisms," *Nature Reviews Cancer* 6, no. 3 (2006): 240–48.

Cohen, Lorenzo, and Alison Jefferies. *Anticancer Living: Transform Your Life and Health with the Mix of Six*. New York: Viking, 2018.

Cunningham, Alastair, and Kimberly Watson. "How Psychological Therapy May Prolong Survival in Cancer Patients: New Evidence and a Simple Theory," *Integrative Cancer Therapies* 3, no. 3 (2004): 214–29.

Dhabhar, Firdaus, et al. "Effect of Stress on Immune Function: The Good, the Bad, and the Beautiful," *Immunologic Research* 58 (2014): 193–210.

Glaser, Ronald, and Janice Kiecolt-Glaser. "Stress-Induced Immune Dysfunction: Implications for Health," *Nature Reviews Immunology* 5, no. 3 (2005): 243–51.

Haus, Erhard, and Michael Smolensky. "Biologic Rhythms in the Immune System," *Chronobiology International* 16, no. 5 (1999): 581–622.

Hauser, David, and Norbert Schwarz. "The War on Prevention: Bellicose Cancer Metaphors Hurt (Some) Prevention Intentions," *Personality & Social Psychology Bulletin* 41, no. 1 (2015): 66–77.

Hong, Suzi, et al. "Effects of Regular Exercise on Lymphocyte Subsets and CD62L After Psychological vs. Physical Stress," *Journal of Psychosomatic Research* 56, no. 3 (2004): 363–70.

Hughes, Spenser, et al. "Social Support Predicts Inflammation, Pain, and Depressive Symptoms: Longitudinal Relationships Among Breast Cancer Survivors," *Psychoneuroendocrinology* 42 (2014): 38–44.

Lerner, Michael. "Difference Between Healing and Curing." *Awakin Readings*. Accessed February 2021. awakin.org/read/view.php ?tid=1066.

Levy, S., et al. "Correlation of Stress Factors with Sustained Depression of Natural Killer Cell Activity and Predicted Prognosis in Patients with Breast Cancer," *Journal of Clinical Oncology* 5, no. 3 (1987): 348–53.

Lutgendorf, S., et al. "Social Influences on Clinical Outcomes of Patients with Ovarian Cancer," *Journal of Clinical Oncology* 30, no. 23 (2012): 2885–90.

Lutgendorf, Susan, et al. "Social Support, Psychological Distress, and Natural Killer Cell Activity in Ovarian Cancer," *Journal of Clinical Oncology* 23, no. 28 (2005): 7105–13.

Pert, Candace, and Nancy Marriot. *Everything You Need to Know to Feel Go(o)d*. Carlsbad: Hay House, 2006.

Raison, Charles, et al. "Cytokines Sing the Blues: Inflammation and the Pathogenesis of Depression," *Trends Immunology* 27, no. 1 (2006): 24–31.

Segertrom, Suzanne, and Gregory Miller. "Psychological Stress and the Human Immune System: A Meta-Analytic Study of 30 Years of Inquiry," *Psychological Bulletin* 130, no. 4 (2004): 601–30.

Witek-Janusek, Linda, et al. "Effect of Mindfulness Based Stress Reduction on Immune Function, Quality of Life and Coping in Women Newly Diagnosed with Early Stage Breast Cancer," *Brain, Behavior, and Immunity* 22, no. 6 (2008): 969–81.

Chapter 8

Besedovsky, Luciana, et al. "Sleep and Immune Function," *Pflügers Archiv: European Journal of Physiology* 463, no. 1 (2012): 121–37.

Sears, William, and Vincent M. Fortanasce. *The Healthy Brain Book: An All-Ages Guide to a Calmer, Happier, Sharper You.* Dallas: BenBella Books, 2020.

Walker, Matthew. *Why We Sleep: Unlocking the Power of Sleep and Dreams.* New York: Scribner, 2017.

Chapter 9

Carlisle, Alison, and N. C. C. Sharp. "Exercise and Outdoor Ambient Air Pollution," *British Journal of Sports Medicine* 35, no. 4 (2001): 214–22.

Curl, Cynthia, et al. "Organophosphorus Pesticide Exposure of Urban and Suburban Preschool Children with Organic and Conventional Diets," *Environmental Health Perspectives* 111, no. 3 (2003): 377–82.

Dean, Amy, and Jennifer Armstrong. "Genetically Modified Foods." *American Academy of Environmental Medicine.* 8 May 2009. aaemonline .org/genetically-modified-foods.

Ellis, K. A., et al. "Comparing the Fatty Acid Composition of Organic and Conventional Milk," *Journal of Dairy Science* 89, no. 6 (2006): 1938–50.

Genuis, Stephen, et al. "Blood, Urine, and Sweat (BUS) Study: Monitoring and Elimination of Bioaccumulated Toxic Elements," *Archives of Environmental Contamination and Toxicology* 61, no. 2 (2011): 344–57.

Grandjean, Philippe, et al. "Serum Vaccine Antibody Concentrations in Children Exposed to Perfluorinated Compounds," *JAMA* 307, no. 4 (2012): 391–97.

Lu, Chensheng, et al. "Organic Diets Significantly Lower Children's Dietary Exposure to Organophosphorus Pesticides," *Environmental Health Perspectives* 114, no. 2 (2006): 260–63.

Mann, Denise. "Childhood Leukemia, Brain Cancer on the Rise." *MedicineNet.* 26 Jan. 2011. medicinenet.com/script/main/art.asp ?articlekey=125152.

"Red Meat and Colon Cancer." *Harvard Health Publishing.* 1 Jan. 2008. health.harvard. edu/staying-healthy/red-meat-and-colon-cancer.

Schafer, Kristin, et al. "Chemical Trespass: Pesticides in Our Bodies and Corporate Accountability." *Pesticide Action Network of North America.* May 2004. panna.org/ resources/publication-report/chemical-trespass.

Index

About the Authors

William Sears, MD, survivor of colon cancer and leukemia, has been advising busy parents on how to raise healthier families for over fifty years and now turns his attention to the specialty of lifestyle medicine. He has served as a voluntary professor at the University of Toronto, University of South Carolina, University of Southern California School of Medicine, and University of California Irvine. As a father of eight children, he coached Little League sports for twenty years, and together with his wife Martha has written more than forty books and countless articles on parenting, nutrition, and healthy aging. He serves as a consultant for TV, magazines, radio, and other media, and his website AskDrSears.com is one of the most popular health and parenting sites. Dr. Sears and his contribution to family health were featured on the cover of *TIME* magazine in May 2012. He is noted for his science-made-simple-and-fun approach to family health and is cofounder of the Dr. Sears Wellness Institute, which has certified over 12,000 health coaches in twenty-two countries.

Martha Sears, RN, is a breast cancer survivor, mother of their eight children, and co-healer in this book.